PROBABILITY

WITHOUT

EQUATIONS

PROBABILITY WITHOUT EQUATIONS

Concepts for Clinicians

BART K. HOLLAND

Division of Biostatistics and Epidemiology
Department of Preventive Medicine
New Jersey Medical School
Newark, New Jersey

The Johns Hopkins University Press

Baltimore and London

© 1998 The Johns Hopkins University Press
All rights reserved. Published 1998
Printed in the United States of America on acid-free paper
07 06 05 04 03 02 01 00 99 98   5 4 3 2 1

The Johns Hopkins University Press
2715 North Charles Street
Baltimore, Maryland 21218-4319
The Johns Hopkins Press Ltd., London

Library of Congress Cataloging-in-Publication Data
will be found at the end of this book.

A catalog record for this book is available from the British Library.

Illustrations on pp. 4, 12, 18, 27, 42, 48, and 62
by Stanley Von Hagen, Ph.D.

ISBN 0-8018-5759-7   ISBN 0-8018-5760-0 (pbk.)

Contents

Contents

Acknowledgments

I owe much to the students of the New Jersey Medical School. Thanks to their questions and comments during the dozen years I have taught there, I have developed and refined the lectures on which this book is based. I appreciate the encouragement of Donald B. Louria, M.D., the chair of the Department of Preventive Medicine at the New Jersey Medical School, who felt that writing this book was a worthwhile effort. I also want to thank Brian Holland for his meticulous reading of the manuscript and his many thoughtful suggestions. My family, of course, has been very supportive.

In a sense, this is a work of translation, for I seek to make the language and thought of the probabilist and statistician accessible to the physician. Some things will necessarily be lost in translation and thus be pronounced inaccurate by the probabilist or uninterpretable by the physician (or both!). It has been said that all translation is a crime against both author and reader. Any errors in this book are entirely my own responsibility. I would appreciate having them brought to my attention, but I would hope that the kind reader will not be too harsh a judge.

PROBABILITY

WITHOUT

EQUATIONS

Introduction

Probability, Uncertainty, and Medical Knowledge

The Nobel prize–winning physicist Ernest Rutherford was fond of saying that if you need statistics to analyze the results of an experiment, you don't have a very good experiment. In a way he was right. However, a recurrent problem in medicine is that in a certain sense you commonly don't have a good experiment—but not because medical research scientists are generally incompetent. The data they work with are simply not as predictable as the data in some other fields, so the predictive value of findings in medical science is generally rather imperfect.

In physics, one may calculate the path of a projectile in advance of its flight. Every time a projectile is launched with the same characteristics, such as starting point, mass, shape, friction, and force, its path will be predictable. It will theoretically follow the same trajectory and end up at the same spot after traveling for the same period of time.

In medicine, things are much less predictable. Two millennia ago, the Roman physician Celsus wrote, "Non omnibus aegris eadem auxilia conveniunt": "The same medicine does not cure every patient." This fact is expressed today when physicians say, "Every patient is different." Indeed, every patient is different, but all patients are still subject to the same physical, chemical, and biological laws. The reason for patient-to-patient variability is that there are countless different variables acting on the patient, some with major and some with minor effects, some interacting synergistically, and some counteracting one another. Some variables are unknown, some unmeasured, some unmeasurable.

With such numerous forces acting on the patient, it is impossible to predict with absolute certainty what will happen to a particular patient. Usually scientists restrict their study to one component of a complex system, and this study may reveal something that is clinically important. For example, the effects of ion concentrations in vitro on aortic tissue may show the importance of certain substances on vasoconstriction, and important insight may thus be gained into an element of vascular disease. In principle, when influences on health are numerous and the effects of any one influence are small, little can be done in the way of intervention.

Prediction and treatment become possible when a few specific factors are of outstanding importance in their effects on health. For example, there are many influences on the occurrence of stroke. Some are genetic factors having to do with the details of the cerebral vasculature. Some factors may be dietary, and they may interact with genetic factors. Social factors, too, may independently affect the risk of stroke, and they are also determinants of, for example, dietary factors. Despite the multiplicity of factors and subfactors and their interactions, reduction of blood pressure through pharmacological intervention is a powerful tool for the reduction of risk of stroke. It remains impossible to predict what will happen with one particular patient, because of the multiplicity of factors affecting him or her and the impossibility of knowing and measuring all of them and assessing their impacts. The effects of the drug itself are likely to vary from person to person, influencing and being influenced by all the factors related to health. Still, biological regularities emerge when we examine masses of people. A large group of people on antihypertensive medication has a lower rate of cerebrovascular hemorrhage than does a group more or less closely matched on other factors but not taking the medication.

So you see that the effects of a treatment (or a particular predictive factor) may be so large as to swamp the effects of other influences on health, and some loosely predictive "law" of therapeutic importance may emerge. In fact, there is a gradient, of course: at one extreme are the diseases for which no known risk factor or treatment has much predictive value, and at the other extreme are diseases for which the interindividual variability in personal, social, biological, or other variables is inconsequential compared to the overwhelming effects of a particular factor. This is sometimes referred to as a gradient in the ratio of "explained variability" to "unexplained variability." The label "explained variability" is attached to differences in outcome between groups who have been classified as to the presence or absence of a risk factor or a therapeutic intervention. The label "unexplained variability" is applied to all other sources of interindividual differences in the outcome.

Unexplained variability is sometimes called "random variation," or the effects of chance. It is not clear that unexplained variability is really random in the sense of being "inherently unpredictable in principle" (the definition of "random" used in today's theories of quantum mechanics); it may instead be variability associated with very many variables, each of which has a tiny effect by itself and perhaps many interactions, so that we cannot know them in detail. Collectively, these many little effects that throw off our prediction are called "error." Chance, in this framework, is merely a measure of our ignorance. Perhaps, as Petronius said, "Suam habet fortuna ratione": "Chance has her own reasons." Anyway, at a certain point in our always-imperfect human knowledge, it essentially *looks* as if there is no material explanation other than chance or random variability for certain effects.

What is important in this situation is the ratio of explained to unexplained variability. When this ratio is low, as it is for some cancers, it means there are no known useful predictive risk factors and no effective treatments as yet. The occurrence of cardiovascular disease in connection with certain risk factors is a cardinal example that makes

---

Explained and Unexplained Variability

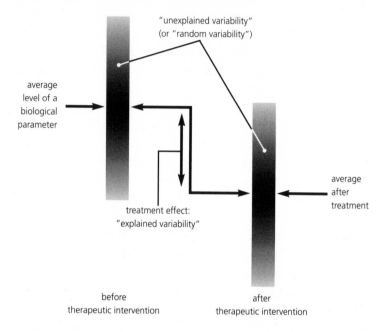

No biological parameter, such as blood pressure, is the same from individual to individual or from day to day within a given patient. In the absence of any therapeutic intervention, a biological parameter has some characteristic level (an average or mean level) and also some variability associated with it, that is, a characteristic spread of values around that mean. After a therapeutic intervention takes place, we hope that a medically useful shift in the mean value of the parameter occurs. This shift is the difference between the *before* and *after* mean values; it's attributed to the treatment effect and is called *explained variability*. Of course, variability not attributed to the therapy still remains. It's unaccounted for by any specific factor or intervention and is called *unexplained variability* or *random variability*.

it abundantly clear that reasoning about disease causality and treatment is an inherently probabilistic exercise: useful, but dicey. On the other hand, the ratio of explained to unexplained variability may be high, meaning that a measurement or a treatment is really very well correlated with the outcome; other factors are of vastly less importance. For example, if a patient has streptococcal septicemia and receives timely treatment with a suitable antibiotic for a sensitive organism, the outcome for the patient may be predicted with a high degree of certainty.

Not perfect certainty, of course. Perhaps the patient has been weakened by other conditions, has an immune abnormality, has come for treatment too late given his or her constitution, or is subject to other chance influences on survival. All diagnoses, treatments, and prognoses are inherently probabilistic, because of the multifactorial nature of influences on human health. So it *is* true that every patient is different and a clinical course is impossible to predict with certainty, and it is equally true that the outcomes in different treatment groups or risk groups exhibit statistical regularities and prediction gets better and better as the sample size increases and these regularities emerge.

Actually, all science dealing with cause-and-effect relations has the problem that its predictive force is vitiated to some degree by random variability. To return to the prediction of trajectories, it must be said that no two objects are ever really identical and have exactly the same trajectories, and no two throws of the same object are exactly the same, even if propelled by machine. Tiny air currents, heat, and other energy effects on the object may have their effects on trajectories too, and all observers make measurement error, no matter how minuscule, in tracking the object. The equations predicting trajectories represent a theoretical path in a perfect situation, never achieved; the equations are correct *on average*, because random effects cancel out. As Gauss showed, the mean of reported locations may be thought of as the true position, because an unbiased measurement taken by an unbiased observer is just as likely to be slightly above as slightly below the true value. And while two manufactured projectiles are unlikely to have exactly the same number of atoms and to be of the same mass, the next one in the shipment is just as likely to have a bit more as to have a bit less mass.

So was Rutherford right? In a sense he was lucky that he was doing certain physics experiments in which random effects could be ignored: they were minimal effects that balanced out. Perhaps in medicine you never (or rarely) have a good experiment, if you insist on defining a good experiment as one elucidating a principle with only inconsequential random variability. However, in studying the determinants of disease and health we are perforce studying a complex system in which many effects of interest are striking, but each may be only part of the story. Many experiments in this field will elucidate scientific facts that will be of practical importance, and intellectually rigorous, as long as we're prepared to accept that in some things probabilistic reasoning is the only avenue to material knowledge open to us, because of the nature of nature. The curative vaccine for rabies, which has near-perfect curative power, is a rarity in medicine, because most medical progress is made in small increments. Modern medical scientists have come to understand the necessity of reasoning probabilistically about many therapies, such as radiation therapy in Hodgkin's lymphoma, the surgical replacement of defective heart valves, or even the use of seatbelts. An understanding that probability is one of the foundations of medical knowledge has stimulated the development of ways of assessing whether an experiment is well designed and statistically valid and has permitted the creation of new therapies whose very real utility could not have been validated without statistical techniques.

One

The Meaning of "Tests of Significance"

What Is a *P* Value?

The students in my medical school classes will no longer gamble with me. They don't trust me, it seems. On the first day of class I repeatedly toss a coin in the air and ask a student to call out to the class, each time, whether the coin ended up heads or tails. As the experiment continues, the sequence of results is rather curious: it consists entirely of heads, one after the other. After a while, someone in the lecture hall inevitably calls out, "It's a fake coin" or "Let us look at the coin" or (worse) "He's cheating." As the experiment progresses, more and more students become convinced that the coin either is a fake coin with two heads or is weighted in some way that it will come up heads no matter how many times it is tossed. Eventually, nearly every student adopts this position, though some hold out for very many tosses. I don't let the students have a good look at the coin. They merely conclude from the unlikely sequence of events that it must be an unfair coin, but they don't *know* that the coin has two heads in the way *I* know it has two heads. They are judging or inferring from the probability of what they have just seen (25 heads in a row, for example) that such an event is so unlikely by chance alone that there must be a better explanation than "it just happened" 25 times in a row. An alternative explanation—that the coin does not have the properties we usually expect of a coin—is more appealing.

The principal features of formal hypothesis testing, as it is practiced in current medical research, are illustrated by this experiment. At any point in the experiment, it is possible to calculate the probability of the observed sequence. Notice that this value can be calculated only if you make certain assumptions. If you think that the chance of getting 25 heads in a row is $(1/2)^{25}$, that is because in doing your calculation you're operating under the assumption that the coin is an ordinary coin that gives a 50-50 chance of turning up either heads or tails. In other words, the probability must be calculated under the assumption that the null hypothesis is true. The *null hypothesis* is the hypothesis of "no difference," the hypothesis that there is nothing special going on and that our usual expectations are met: there is nothing special or different about that coin. If what we observe is so improbable as to strain credulity, we say that the data do not support the null hypothesis and that we will accept an *alternative hypothesis* as more likely.

That is the logic of hypothesis testing in clinical trials and epidemiological studies, among other areas of medical research. In clinical trials, the null hypothesis might be that two drugs do not differ in their pharmacological effectiveness or that a new drug is indistinguishable from a placebo in its therapeutic effects. In an epidemiological study, the null hypothesis might be that people who live near high-voltage electric lines do not have an elevated risk of certain cancers. The mechanics of the computations may be complicated, but the principle remains the same: we calculate the probability of seeing a given difference in the proportion of patients improving, by chance alone, when on average there is no difference. Or we may calculate the probability that not one, but two or three or five members of a family living near high-tension wires would all happen to be patients with a certain cancer. And then we judge whether the probability that this could have occurred under the null hypothesis offends our sense of what is reasonably likely.

The concept of "reasonably likely" is an arbitrary one. Some students in my classes question whether the coin is genuine very early in the experiment, when it has turned up heads just a few times; others wait and see and finally come to believe the coin is a fake only after many tosses. These students have different internal criteria for what is too unlikely by chance alone to be acceptable. In statistical terminology, they have different *alpha* (or α) *levels.* The arbitrary nature of the alpha level must be clearly understood. No student has an "incorrect" alpha level when deciding to accept that the coin must be fake. Some students have a more rigid criterion, whereas others are quick to draw a conclusion. There is no objective rule that gives us a reason to choose one alpha level over another.

The alpha level should not be confused with the *P* value. The *P* value is calculated from data. It tells you the probability that a set of observations as extreme as or more extreme than those actually observed would happen by chance alone. It is the chance that you would actually observe certain freakish data sets as the outcome of your experiment, given that the null hypothesis is true. The expression "as extreme as or more extreme than" is used because the chance of obtaining any given set of data—10 specific systolic blood pressures, for example—is extremely small, even if it's the chance of getting 10 observations of exactly the mean blood pressure for a group. So unlikely outcomes are bundled together, and probabilities are calculated for data in a range "as extreme as or more extreme than" than the observed data. The alpha level is also a probability, but it is a preset criterion level of probability. If *P* is less than alpha, the null hypothesis is considered unsupported by the data, and the finding is considered *statistically significant.*

In medical research it is common to accept that interesting findings did not happen by chance if the probability of the observations is less than 0.05, less than 0.01, or less than 0.001. This means that if the null hypothesis were in fact true, you'd see such an extreme set of observations (or a more extreme set of observations) less than 5%, less than 1%, or less than one-tenth of 1% of the time. If you read the medical journals, you are well aware that these three choices of alpha level are used in the vast majority of research. The reason for this prevalence is a historical one: early in the twentieth century, before the use of calculators or computers, there was a need for published tables that would permit the assessment of the rarity of particular sequences of events. An impractically voluminous publication would have resulted if a *P* value had been shown for every conceivable case

Pizza Cures Chicken Pox . . . or Does It?

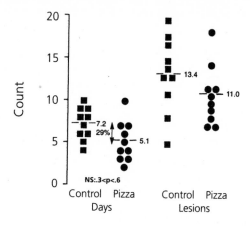

Sampling fluctuation is one reason that two samples may have different mean values, even if they're both drawn from populations that are identical with respect to the measured characteristic. Suppose that eating pizza has no bearing on the course of disease in chickenpox patients; it affects neither the number of days of illness nor the number of lesions. In the data shown in the figure above, which were actually collected, the mean number of days of illness is 29% higher in chickenpox patients who did not eat pizza than in those who did (7.2 days versus 5.1 days). The mean number of lesions is also different (13.4 versus 11.0). But modest differences like these are likely to occur by chance alone, given these sample sizes, even in two samples drawn from a population with mean values in common. The probability of observing such differences in samples drawn by chance is between 0.3 and 0.6, or in the neighborhood of 50-50. This means the findings are not surprising and hence are not statistically significant.

Source: Thomas E. Bradstreet, "Teaching Introductory Statistics Courses so that Nonstatisticians Experience Statistical Reasoning," *American Statistician*, *50*, no. 1 (1996): 74. Reprinted with permission of *American Statistician*. Copyright 1996 by the American Statistical Association.

of, for example, proportions of therapeutic successes seen when comparing two treatment groups. So tables were drawn up and published showing, for instance, the ratios of success rates (standardized for sample size) that corresponded to a few "round" values of probabilities of occurrence. Such tables presented a few arbitrary probabilities, chosen by a renowned statistician named Ronald Fisher, and the observed measurement that would correspond to each arbitrary level of rarity. If an experimenter had a set of observations more extreme than that which marked the boundary at $\alpha = 0.05$ but less extreme than that required for $\alpha = 0.01$, the probability of the set of observations was in between these two P values. The observations were said to be statistically significant at $\alpha = 0.05$ but not at $\alpha = 0.01$. Much subsequent statistical work aped these few choices for alpha, and since people have become familiar with them, they have remained of key importance in statistics even though computers now allow much flexibility in the calculation of probabilities. If you were to submit an article to a medical journal and wrote that "our decision criterion for statistical significance was an alpha level preset at 0.03 [or, say, 0.007]," the journal's editors and referees would most likely ask you to defend your choice of alpha level. Nonetheless, the levels of alpha that are accepted in science are the result of historical accident, namely, a lack of computing facilities combined with practical pressures and what seemed sensible to Ronald Fisher.

Possible Errors in Hypothesis Testing

There is another way to look at alpha level. It is not only a decision criterion, but also the quantification of an acceptable error rate, at least under a certain circumstance. Suppose that the null hypothesis that a new drug gives a 50-50 chance of cure is true but we don't know this, and in our first observations of the drug's effects we witness 10 successes in a row. The chance of that happening is small (0.5^{10} is less than one chance in a thousand), but it will occur by chance alone in a known proportion of possible trials even when the

Testing a Null Hypothesis

In significance testing, a certain set of assumptions is made, called the *null hypothesis*. Suppose the null hypothesis is that taking a given drug has no antihypertensive effect. Then a sample set of observations is drawn, and the probability of such a set of observations is calculated. The calculation is based on the null hypothesis, together with sampling theory: if the mean antihypertensive effect is in fact zero, and only random fluctuation in systolic blood pressure is occurring, how often would samples of the given size be drawn that end up with lots of high or low values by chance alone, resulting in a mean change so different from zero? The probability of such a difference, or a more extreme difference, by chance alone, occupies a particular zone on the continuum of probabilities shown in the above figure. The more toward the center our calculated probability, the more it's in accord with our expectations, and the further out it is, the less likely it is that the difference is due to sampling fluctuation. At some point, we draw a line and say the finding is too unlikely to be chance alone. When we obtain such a finding, we offer another explanation, different from the null hypothesis. The spot where we draw the line is called *alpha* (or α), and it's an arbitrary probability value, such as 0.05, 0.01, or 0.001. We may also restrict our interest to the rarest values on one or the other side of the null hypothesis value, if big differences in one direction are of clinical interest and differences in the other direction are not. If we consider the probability of sampling fluctuation in only one direction, our test is called *one-tailed*, rather than *two-tailed*.

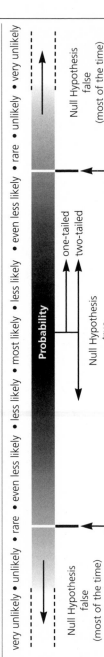

null hypothesis is true. So suppose the decision criterion has been set at, say, 0.05, and the null hypothesis happens to be true (unbeknownst to us). There is then a 5% chance that a set of observations will occur that will be declared statistically significant, even though this declaration is an error. It is an error because a difference from a 50-50 success rate in this case does not actually exist but will be the finding of the hypothesis test. The error rate can be quantified in advance of the experiment: if in fact no difference exists, we will nonetheless say that one exists, 5% of the time. This is called the *alpha error*, or the *Type I error*.

This problem of error is compounded by what is called the *multiple testing problem*. If the alpha level is 0.05 and the null hypothesis is true, the chance of correctly stating after an experiment that "the null hypothesis is true" is 0.95. Suppose in a complex study 20 null hypotheses are tested, and each one is found to be true. The chance of correctly stating that all 20 null hypotheses are true is 0.95^{20} and is therefore equal to 0.3585. This means that it is *more likely than not* that a statistically significant result is found, even though each one is tested at a reasonable level of 0.05 and only chance effects are operating. There are corrections for this, such as Bonferroni's correction, which you'll see referred to in reports of studies in which many hypotheses were tested. In effect, these usually aim at making the alpha level for the overall set of hypotheses conform to the selected alpha value. However, this can make it extremely difficult to detect specific effects, so there's a trade-off.

To think of a distinctly clinical example of the multiple testing problem, note that the normal range of laboratory values for many clinical tests is defined as the range in which 95% of observations from people without disease will lie. This method (or the selection of some other percentage of common values) is the usual way of defining normal ranges in clinical laboratories, because the ranges of observations from normal and diseased patients typically have substantial overlap. People with values outside the normal range, that is, values quite rare in disease-free individuals, may be either diseased or simply normal people with unusual values for that laboratory parameter for chance reasons not related to the pathology under study. A person may have high intraocular pressure without the pathology of glaucoma or low blood sugar with the pathology of diabetes, and the body temperatures of patients with and without infections are described by overlapping bell-shaped curves. So lab work has artificial and arbitrary boundaries, too, because biological measurements usually exist along a continuum; "drawing the line somewhere" is merely a matter of human definition and convenience. A clinical lab report "flagging" some "abnormality" is important information, but often it is only a piece of the clinical picture. However, since many lab testing procedures divide the world of patients into "normal" and "abnormal," and since a certain given proportion of disease-free people will have abnormal test results, the multiple testing problem rears its ugly head. If you order 20 lab tests that were constructed with the normal range defined as "95% of the range of measurement in disease-free people," once again the chance that some lab value from a disease-free person will come back flagged as abnormal by chance alone is 0.3585. So if your patient is normal, the more tests you perform, the more likely it is that something will come back from the lab that reflects an extreme value merely by chance but is marked as a clinically relevant deviation from normality.

Can the multiple testing problem be avoided by setting a much more restrictive alpha level? For example, could we specify that a finding is statistically significant only if it would happen under the null hypothesis by chance alone less than 0.0001 of the time, or even 0.00000001 of the time? Although we can never be absolutely certain that a null hypothesis is untrue, our feeling of certainty gets stronger as the P value gets smaller. One million heads in a row, or a billion heads in a row, clearly offers a probability approaching certainty about the two-headed nature of my coin, especially compared to 10 flips of the coin. So there would be a great advantage in that way. However, there is a disadvantage to using overly strict alpha levels. To demonstrate a one-in-a-million finding would take a long time. If that were some of my students' criterion for decision making, a minute or two of coin tossing wouldn't permit a definitive experiment to determine the fairness of my coin. Perhaps a clinical study with very many patients would be too expensive to organize and follow through and would take too long to complete in view of the need to find a solution to the clinical problem in the short term. What usually happens is a compromise. A study must be of a practical size, and in statistical terms it must achieve an experimenter-defined "reasonable balance" between the two possible types of statistical error, which are shown in Table 1.

Table 1
Possible Errors in Hypothesis Testing

		The TRUTH is . . .	
		H_0	H_A
You say . . .			
	H_0	no problem	Type II (ß) error
	H_A	Type I (α) error	no problem

Note: H_0, the null hypothesis; H_A, the alternative hypothesis.

There are two happy situations in which no errors occur. If in truth the null hypothesis ought to be accepted and you say that it is true based on your experimental findings, or if in fact some alternative hypothesis holds and you correctly infer from your experiment that this is the case, then there has been no error. The first type of error that may occur in hypothesis testing is alpha error, or Type I error, which we already know is the chance of declaring that a significant difference exists, given that the null hypothesis is true. The second type of error is *beta error* (β), or *Type II error*. This is the chance that you fail to detect a difference that in fact exists, so that you erroneously declare the null hypothesis to be true.

Statistical Power

Beta error has just been defined as the probability that you fail to detect an existing difference. Its complement, $1 - ß$, is the probability that you *do* detect the existing difference, and this is the definition of statistical power.

There is an important and complex interplay between alpha and beta errors, sample size, and statistical power in medical studies. The coin toss example will illustrate this. We've already reviewed what alpha error is by using a demonstration based on my tossing a two-headed coin. It is clear from that demonstration that as the specified value of alpha gets smaller and smaller it becomes necessary to have a larger and larger sample size (number of coin tosses) to establish proof of a difference. Also, as the sample size increases, if we hold alpha constant, it becomes possible to detect a smaller and smaller difference that may exist between the values specified in the null and alternative hypotheses. For example, if, instead of a two-headed coin, I have one that is simply weighted so that it comes up heads 60% of the time, it will take longer to reach some specified alpha level. For a coin weighted so that it turns up heads 52% of the time, a very large sample size indeed would be needed. Thus, statistical power (1 − beta error rate) goes up with increasing sample size and with increasing difference existing in the system, given that the alternative hypothesis is true. Finally, alpha and beta error rates move in opposite directions. That is, assuming some fixed combination of sample size and existing difference, if an investigator picks a higher value of alpha (0.05 rather than 0.0001, for example), then beta will be lowered and statistical power, or 1 − ß, will increase.

Sample size is of great practical importance in clinical research. Most experiments involve considerable amounts of logistical planning, expense, and time, because they require that patients, animals, or cultures be accrued and clinical or lab information on them be obtained. Personnel and materials must be committed, and people are often waiting with interest for the outcomes, which may have considerable clinical significance. So sample size is usually set in advance for planning purposes.

Sample size is determined by a set of trade-offs, because it is desirable to avoid a sample size that is either too large or too small. A large sample size is useful in allowing small but clinically meaningful effects to be detected if they are present, but it is wasteful if effects are not present. It is also wasteful to have pursued a very large sample if it turns out that sought-after clinical differences are larger than expected, but usually an experiment can be stopped earlier than expected if massive effects are seen. In fact, there is an ethical reason to interrupt a study that achieves statistical significance early, because once the new information has been established no one should be subjected to experimentation that was originally designed to obtain that information. In addition, if there is an implication for treatment, treatment plans should then be altered early to incorporate what has been learned.

Even from the start, to envision too large a sample size is counterproductive. If the sample size were huge enough, any difference could be detected and declared to be statistically significant, for example, even a one-tenth of 1% improvement in the therapeutic success rate. There is really no point to having a sample size large enough to demonstrate the statistical significance of a difference that has no clinical significance.

Too small a sample size is also undesirable, as is a bit more obvious. Two or three tosses of a coin would not suffice to let you determine whether I'm using a two-headed coin. To pick a more clinically relevant example, suppose a drug company claims that a certain medication provides an 80% therapeutic success rate for patients with a given condition. You have three patients in your practice with that condition, but only one is a therapeutic success with that medication. Is one out of three a surprising finding if the null hypothesis of an 80% success rate is true? Does the finding lead you to suspect the company of misrepresenting the therapeutic success rate? Or is the difference between your observed rate and the rate specified by the null hypothesis reasonable to expect by chance alone? It turns out that the P value in that situation is 0.096, and so it is nearly 10% of the time that only one out of three would be therapeutic successes.

In good scientific investigations, sample size is usually set jointly

Determinants of Statistical Power

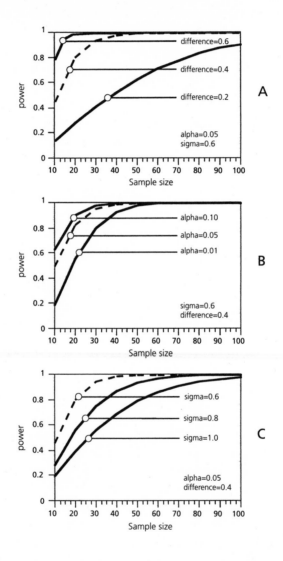

Statistical power depends on several factors: the alpha level of the statistical test, the sample size used, the difference to be detected, and the variability of the measured variable. The importance of each of these factors can be understood by examining the above figure, which varies them one at a time while holding the others constant.

In panel A, alpha is kept at 0.05, and sigma (the standard deviation) is also arbitrarily kept at a particular value, 0.6. The infinite possible patterns of differences between group means are represented by three varying values: 0.6, 0.4, and 0.2. (Technically, these three values are called *mean squared differences* because for each of the observations in a group, the differences from a specified value are measured, squared, and summed, and then an average value is taken for that set of observations). Notice that as the difference gets larger, greater statistical power can be achieved with the same sample size.

In panel B, sigma is again kept constant at the arbitrary value of 0.6, and now the difference is held constant, too, at 0.4. Alpha varies between three different levels. As the desired alpha level gets more stringent, statistical power diminishes for a given sample size. One must increase the sample size to maintain a given level of statistical power as one goes to stricter (smaller) alpha levels.

In panel C, the alpha and the difference are kept constant, and sigma varies. As the standard deviation increases, statistical power decreases, because if a parameter has a lot of inherent variability it's more difficult to distinguish a difference between groups from that inherent variability. One may have to increase the sample size to maintain a desired statistical power.

by the investigator and a biostatistician. The calculation may be simple or may be complex and done by computer, but it always involves certain elements. First, the investigator decides on the variable(s) that will be studied and the criterion for the size of a clinically meaningful difference. Next, an alpha level is set in consultation with the statistician: will it be acceptable to run a 5% risk that a difference is called significant when in fact none exists? Or will some stricter ("more conservative") alpha level be used, such as 0.001? Usually, if the effects being postulated seem to be biologically implausible, go against accepted wisdom, or would have great reverberations in the world of science or medicine, more conservative alpha levels are picked—this lessens the chance of going off half-cocked, declaring a remarkable finding that later cannot be replicated because it was never there in the first place. Finally, the certainty of detection of an expected finding is jointly decided on: this is statistical power of the study. Based on the specification of alpha, the statistical power, the difference to be detected, and the statistical test to be used, the sample size is calculated using various formulas, usually by the biostatistician.

Sometimes this sequence is altered a bit because of practical considerations, such as a marked limit to patient accrual or the availability of only a limited number of specimens. In such cases, the statistician works backward, starting with the sample size, and can tell an investigator what can be achieved in the way of statistical power given various choices of alpha and various postulated effect sizes. Sometimes the statistician determines that there can be no reasonable expectation that the experiment will be able to demonstrate anything of statistical significance, because the sample size is too small, given the effect postulated, to detect clinically interesting effects and establish that they're not likely by chance. This is important, if unwelcome, advice. Why waste resources on an experiment that most likely will not be adequate to show the effects of interest? Moreover, it is unethical to carry out an experiment on people (or animals) that does not have a reasonable prospect of success.

Two

Alphabet Soup

t, Z, F, r, and Other Statistics Found in the Medical Literature

The Concepts of Distribution and Sample

If you calculate the chance of getting 25 heads in a row when tossing a fair coin as 0.5^{25}, you may not be aware of it but you make a number of statistical assumptions because of your intuitive understanding of the probabilistic aspects of the situation. In fact, calculating the probability would have been impossible without making those assumptions. The first, obvious assumption you make is that only heads or tails can occur and that one of the two must occur. No missing data allowed, and no landing on edges or rolling away.

Less obvious is the assumption of statistical independence, which is the assumption that what happens on one coin toss has no bearing on what happens on the next. With a fair coin this is true, so it is an appropriate assumption to make when calculating probabilities under the null hypothesis. With a biased coin or two-headed coin this is not true, because if you know the bias of the coin, one guess is *not* as good as the other in terms of predicting the next outcome. The assumption of independence is almost always an important assumption in medical statistics. A group is assumed to be a random sample of patients; that is, it is assumed that what happens with one patient has no bearing on what happens with the next. In a study designed to measure the results of the anticoagulant warfarin, the effects of warfarin would be incorrectly assessed if all the patients came from a family with a rare genetic absence of the receptor for warfarin, in whom only enormous doses of warfarin have any measurable physiological effect. A few such families actually exist. In a large random sample, with independent selection of cases, you'll get, on average, a representative group of people whose medical histories and outcomes have no bearing on one another. In comparisons of two or more groups of patients, there is a great advantage to randomly allocating patients to the groups, rather than putting, for example, all friends, relatives, and family members into a group or all patients from similar clinics with similar histories into a group. The advantage is that, on average, high- and low-risk patients end up more or less equally distributed in the groups. The larger the sample size and the more perfectly random the allocation, the more truly comparable the groups will be. And this comparability is required for the validity of P values from hypothesis tests.

Another important assumption for the calculation of P values is that the observations correspond to a random sample *from some particular distribution.* A probability distribution may be conceived of as a list of possible outcomes, with the probability of each specified. In the case of the coin toss experiment, we assume that the outcomes can be modeled by the *binomial* distribution. Sometimes this can be calculated quite easily; most people can calculate the probability of getting two heads in a row when tossing a coin. However, sometimes a mathematical equation makes it easier or is required. For example, it is not an easy matter to figure out the probability of observing 57 heads out of 10,000 coin tosses, even though you know it is a low probability. In the equations, certain parameters are required. For example, with the binomial distribution, you need to plug in the number of tosses, the chance of getting heads on each toss, and the number of heads actually observed. With these "knowns" entered, you can perform the arithmetic operations prescribed by the formula and determine the P value.

There are many distributions of great use in medical statistics, and they're usually more complicated mathematically than the binomial or other simple categorical formulations. A very common continuous distribution is the bell-shaped curve called the *Gaussian distribution,* or *normal distribution.* Many biological measurements, such as blood pressure, height, weight, birth weight, physiological response to many drugs, circulating hormone levels, circulating antibody levels, and many more, are empirically well described by the normal distribution. If we can accept the assumption that a variable is normally distributed, we can plug two parameters into the mathematical formula for the normal distribution: the *mean* of the observations and the *standard deviation,* a summary measure of the observations' variation from the mean. With these in the equation, together with any one particular observation value, arithmetic calculation allows us to obtain the probability that corresponds to that particular observation. As usual, if it is too rare by our alpha criterion we will declare that the small *P* value demonstrates statistical significance. This is called a *Z test.*

Sampling Variability and Statistical Tests

With many variables in biology and medicine, the outcome is not a discrete binary variable such as heads/tails, cured/not cured, but instead is a continuous measurement, such as blood pressure, blood cell count, lung capacity, or the range of motion of a joint. These data are described by continuous distributions such as the normal distribution mentioned in the previous section. Measurement data obviously have variability associated with them. (So do data such as coin toss outcomes, but the calculation of that variability is more straightforward than for measurement data.) Some of the variability in physiological measurements is "noise" or "junk" variability, without any clinical significance. For example, the same instrument in the same lab may give a slightly different blood cell count when a specimen is rerun through it by the same technician who ran the specimen through it the first time. Within one person there is another source of variability: random variation, again of no significance. If blood is drawn from the same disease-free, infection-free individual at the same time of day for 2 or 3 days in a row, blood cell counts as determined by flow cytometry may vary substantially.

The variation we care about in medical research is nonrandom variation, that is, variation associated with factors of diagnostic or therapeutic significance. Flow cytometry results may differ considerably between HIV-infected and uninfected patients and between HIV-infected patients who are receiving drug treatment and those who are not. Flow cytometry results may be an extremely useful tool for prognosis in these groups of patients, but to assess the differences between groups we need to be able to distinguish variability associated with group membership from other variability we don't care about. In terminology borrowed from radio engineering, this latter type of variability is called *noise,* and the observed differences that we care about are called the *signal.*

The *signal-to-noise ratio* is crucial to our ability to detect meaningful differences between groups under study. If the data are very noisy, meaning that they include a lot of random variation, it will be very difficult to detect a weak signal. For example, if random variation in a cell count were 1,000 from one blood drawing to the next, but a drug we're working on has the reliable and reproducible physiological effect of increasing that cell count by 500, it may not be possible to distinguish that very real but modest effect from random variation. As the strength of the signal increases relative to the random variation, it becomes more likely that the effect will be detected: statistical power increases.

Often the "observation" we wish to plug into the equation for a distribution is actually a mean value, such as blood pressure, for a sample, because it is impractical to take lab measurements on every patient with a given condition. Thus, there is an additional source of variability introduced. This source of variability is called *sampling error.* It exists because when a value is estimated from a sample, that estimate will vary somewhat from the true mean in the population from which the sample is drawn, because of the luck of the draw as to who gets selected.

This sampling variability follows a regular, provable law called the *central limit theorem,* which says that sample means, if actually drawn at random, are just as likely to be a bit above as a bit below the mean of the population they represent. So there is a distribution of sample means, and on average a sample mean is an unbiased estimator of the true population mean. The mean of sample means ultimately yields the population mean, and this is increasingly true as the sizes of samples increase and as the number of samples increases. The additional variability due to sampling must be factored in when calculating *P* values, however, and is related to the sample size. To estimate mean height in a medical school class of 175 students without taking the trouble to measure them all, I might measure a sample. A sample of 173 will vary little from the overall true population mean. However, a sample of 20 is a less reliable estimator of that population mean, and a sample of 3 is less reliable still, because sampling variability (the luck of the draw) plays an increasing part as sample size decreases. I might get the 3 tallest or shortest people in my sample of 3; such peculiarness is less likely by chance in the sample of 20 and of little importance in the sample of 173.

The *t* Test

The *t* distribution allows us to calculate the probability of seeing particular observations, which come from samples in the form of means or differences between the means of two groups. The formula involves the use of the square root of the sample size to adjust the measure of variability. Dividing the standard deviation by the square root of the sample size provides the *standard error.* Here the standard error is the summary measure of the noise variability, the difference in the mean values is the signal, and the ratio of the signal to the standard error is the *t* statistic. Tables of calculated values are available in books and computer programs that tell you the *t* value that must be achieved with different sample sizes (for a range of alpha levels) before a result can be declared statistically significant. These tables exist because the probability of a particular observed sample can be calculated, given the sample size and the assumption of a mean specified by the null hypothesis. If a population has a certain mean, you can calculate the probability that a sample of a given size will have a different mean. The more different the sample, the less likely it is that it would come from that population. Finally, at some point, a sample might be so peculiar that you feel it is too unlikely to have been drawn from the population of interest, and the null hypothesis is not supported.

An adjustment can be made in the *t* test whereby samples are paired, instead of independent, as in the above example. In paired samples, data are from before-and-after measurements on the same individual, from twins, or from people otherwise quite closely matched on factors affecting the variable under study. For example, in a paired *t* test, the observations might be the changes in blood pressure in a group of people observed before and after long-term treatment with an antihypertensive medication. Each individual serves as his or her own control. This experiment avoids the comparison of blood pressure in one group (taking the drug) with that in a group of controls (not taking the drug).

The advantage of having individuals serve as their own control is that some sources of variability are eliminated. If there were separate drug and control groups, part of the difference between the blood pressures in the two groups would be noise: random variation between persons in the two groups with respect to factors that happen to give them blood pressure a bit higher or lower or affect their response to the drug. With the paired *t* test, interpersonal sources of random fluctuation in blood pressure are eliminated. There is still *intra*personal variability contributing to noise in the system, but there is less random variability overall. Therefore, for a given signal or existing difference, there is an enhanced signal-to-noise ratio, and it is easier to find statistical significance with a paired test at any given sample size than with a test of independent samples with the same number of measurements. In other words, given a particular sam-

Finding Statistically Significant Differences

The factors that make for a statistically significant difference are perhaps best illustrated by one of the simplest and commonest types of hypothesis-testing situations: the attempt to distinguish between the means of two different groups using a *t* test. The attempt will be successful if the magnitude of the difference is large compared to the variability one typically sees in the type of measurements one is comparing. This is shown in the figure below. In panel A, the blood pressures of treated and untreated patients follow normal frequency distributions with different mean values (called μ_1 and μ_2), and the difference between them is $\mu_1 - \mu_2$. In panel B, the difference between the two groups is exactly the same as in panel A, but the variability in the measurements is less. Since there is therefore less overlap in the two distributions, statistical significance will be easier to detect. In panel C, the variability is the same as in panel A, but a larger difference in the mean values makes it likely that statistical significance will be detected. When clinicians are concerned with differences in mean values and are interested in testing for significance, they're commonly asked by their statistical colleagues to provide estimates of both the difference and the variability in the groups, because calculations of *P* values for many statistical tests are based on these two values.

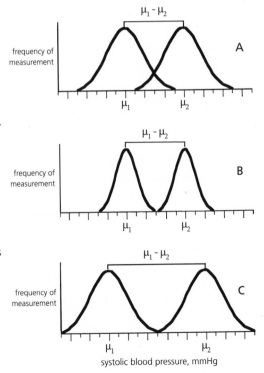

ple size *n*, statistical power is enhanced if the *n* observations are all from one group rather than from two groups. *P* value calculation formulas exist for both the independent and paired cases of *t* tests.

One-Tailed or Two-Tailed Test of Significance?

In the medical journals, it is common to see a distinction made between "one-tailed" and "two-tailed" tests of significance. This is because a sample can be peculiar in one of two directions. For example, in the *t*-test situation, a sample might be a one-in-a-million finding far above the mean value, or it might be a one-in-a-million finding far below the mean. If we're considering only those results far afield in one direction as conflicting with our reasonable expectations and falsifying the null hypothesis, we're performing a one-tailed test. Here's an example of a one-tailed, clinically meaningful alternative hypothesis: "Patients in drug treatment group X have reduced systolic blood pressure after six weeks compared to patients in drug treatment group Y." We're interested in a finding in only one direction, because the comparison of the two groups has clinical relevance in only one direction, assuming that there's no clinical utility for a drug that raises blood pressure. A two-tailed alternative hypothesis would be, "Patients in drug treatment group X are no different with respect to systolic blood pressure after six weeks compared to patients in drug treatment group Y."

As you may suspect, it's easier to find statistical significance in a one-tailed test than in a two-tailed test. Suppose we're using an alpha level of 0.05. Then a finding that would happen only 5% of the time by chance alone is considered a statistically significant difference. In a one-tailed test, the 5% of observations that are most unlikely and are clinically relevant to the hypothesis are either all the highest or all the lowest observations we can get. However, in a two-tailed test, the 5% of the observations that are the least likely include both the 2½% rarest observations on the high end and the 2½% rarest observations on the low end. It's a lot easier to have an observation by chance that would occur 5% of the time than to have one that would occur 2½% of the time, so if we concentrate on one direction and consider the 5% rarest observations of interest to be concentrated all in that direction, we're more likely to declare that a randomly selected sample mean was statistically significant. This is the gain we enjoy for knowing something about what is likely to occur and restricting our hypothesis on this basis.

However, we must decide that we really care about a change in only one direction, test accordingly, and stick with that preset criterion. It is cheating to change the testing format after examining the results. If a two-tailed test is performed with $\alpha = 0.05$, and the observation is among the 3% rarest observations in the high direction, significance will not be reached when the t statistic is compared to the tabled values of t, because the P value does not indicate sufficient rarity. The observation would have to be in the 97.5th percentile, not in the 97th as observed, for the finding to be significant in this scenario. It would be cheating to switch after this finding and say that the findings were significant after all, in a one-tailed test with $\alpha = .05$. It is cheating because it is inappropriate to gain from the experiment previously unknown information as to the direction of the difference and then test as if you had known all along that that would be the direction. If you *had* known all along that the observations would be different in the positive direction, you should have been doing a one-tailed test to begin with.

Analysis of Variance

The *analysis of variance,* often abbreviated *anova,* can be seen as an extension of the t test to three or more groups. A common way to proceed is to look for support for a global alternative hypothesis, such as, "There are differences in systolic blood pressure dependent on membership in treatment categories." An F test is usually used to determine whether the data reflect this or, instead, reflect the null hypothesis of no differences. The F test is most explicitly a test of the signal-to-noise-ratio. The observed value for F is calculated as a ratio: on top is the variability associated with group membership; on the bottom is the variability *within* groups, that is, person-to-person variability that is assumed to be random. Then, specific pairwise comparisons may be made: treatments 1 versus 2, 1 versus 3, and 2 versus 3. The tests for such pairwise comparisons include Bonferroni's and Duncan's tests. These two follow logic analogous to that for the t test.

There are many types of anova, which differ largely in the sampling scheme they include. For example, a sample of clinics may be drawn, and then within each of the clinics a sample of patients may be drawn. This is done in the hopes of obtaining a representation of a large group of people in a convenient way, without having to study every individual. However, this method introduces new sources of sampling variability: there is some error in estimating mean values because not all clinics were selected, and some error in estimating mean values for the selected clinics because not every individual was examined within those clinics. These sources of error are carefully attributed and quantified, and a large literature exists on the elaborate calculations needed to estimate P values in these and other complex anova models.

Another anova design is referred to as *repeated measures anova.* This is somewhat similar to the paired t test in that there are repeated measures on each of the various individuals in a study. These might be before-and-after measurements or a series of sequential measurements, such as body weight among people on various weight loss regimens, head circumferences of babies as they grow during the first year of life, or sequential CD4 counts among patients on various combination therapies for HIV infection. As with the paired t test, there is a gain in power from having each individual serve as his or her own control. For example, if observations are taken at 0, 3, 6, 9, and 12 months of age from each member of a single cohort of infants, and not from five different samples of infants at those five different ages, interinfant variability is eliminated. Thus within-group variability is lessened, and with the noise in the system diminished, existing differences are easier to detect.

Analogous Nonparametric Methods

Hypothesis testing associated with observed *Z, t,* and *F* statistics is predicated on the knowledge of what happens when random samples are drawn in situations governed by the mathematical properties of the normal distribution. This knowledge allows *P* values to be calculated for a wide variety of situations. The central limit theorem demonstrates that all sampling may be governed by this quantitative knowledge. For example, the means of samples of any size, if repeated often enough, will have a normal distribution centered on the population mean, regardless of whether the population from which the samples are drawn follows a normal distribution or not. This fact can be demonstrated mathematically and makes possible such tests as the *t* and *F* tests. However, the fact that the approximation of the true mean by the samples becomes demonstrably, quantifiably better as you get more and more (and bigger and bigger) samples has an important implication: at very small sample sizes, especially samples drawn from distributions far from normal, the approximation of the population value is not yet accurate.

This problem is dealt with by what are called *nonparametric* methods. Nonparametric methods do not require the assumption of the mathematical theory of the probabilities associated with normal distributions. They do not provide *P* values based on areas under a normal curve, which would require knowledge of parameters (mean and standard deviation) for calculation. They do not rely directly on measurements, either, but simply on the rank order, from lowest to highest, of observations in samples.

An easily understood nonparametric test is *Wilcoxon's rank sum test.* It is analogous to a *t* test but is performed on the ranks of the observations, not on the observations themselves (if indeed they are available, which they need not be). To understand this test, consider the experiments presented schematically in Table 2. In experiment 1, a group of patients randomized to drug A are being compared with a group randomized to drug B. In experiment 2, the two patient groups are receiving drugs C and D. Some outcome measure, such as forced expiratory volume or number of asthmatic attacks, is observed. The truth is that drugs A and B are not different, and the outcome in experiment 1 reflects this fact perfectly. The 10 outcomes are ranked from lowest to highest, and the patient with the first outcome is found in drug group A, the second in B, the third in A, the fourth in B, and so on. There is no difference between the treatments, so the ranks are completely interspersed between drug A recipients and drug B recipients. The other extreme obtains in experiment 2. The effects of the two treatments are completely divergent. All 5 lowest values are found in the group receiving drug C, and all 5 highest values are found in the group receiving drug D.

Table 2
Data for Rank Sum Tests

	Experiment 1		*Experiment 2*	
	Drug A	Drug B	Drug C	Drug D
	1	2	1	6
	3	4	2	7
	5	6	3	8
	7	8	4	9
	9	10	5	10
Total	25	30	15	40

Notice that in the interspersed data in experiment 1, the sums of the ranks are 25 and 30, respectively. In the divergent data in experiment 2, since the low values are in one group and the high values in the other, the sums of the ranks are more divergent: 15 and 40. The sum of all whole numbers from 1 to 10 is 55, so the sum of *all* ranks must be 55 for experiment 1 and likewise for experiment 2; indeed, it must be 55 for all experiments with 10 observations. So there is a range of splits that can occur, from 25:30 (no association between drug and outcome) to 15:40 (perfect association). If in fact there is no association, as the splits widen from 25:30 to 15:40 they are less likely to be observed in a sample. Wilcoxon's rank sum test results from mathematical calculations that permit the calculation of P values for the various possible splits, given various possible sample sizes in experiments.

Various refinements to the test have been made, such as a method of allowing for ties (use the average rank between two tied values), but here it is the principle we wish to understand: nonparametric tests can be used when the data set contains just a few observations or when normal distribution calculations are unwarranted, for example, when the data consist only of ranks. Nonparametric analogues for anova exist, and this anova on ranks provides a statistic allowing the examination of P values in what is called the *Kruskal-Wallis test*. Nonparametric tests have also been worked out for a large variety of other situations. Since nonparametric tests use cruder information than parametric tests use, they have distinct advantages and disadvantages. It has already become clear that nonparametric analysis can be used in many situations in which parametric analysis can't, such as experiments that produce a small number of rank order data but not measurements. On the other hand, because they use coarser data there is generally a loss of statistical power in nonparametric tests compared with their parametric counterparts, and small samples are more sensitive to random fluctuations. Thus to guard against a given level of alpha error, differences often must be substantial to be statistically significant.

Chi-Square and Other Methods of Analyzing Categorical Data

Many data in medicine are inherently categorical. For example, a new lab test for the presence or absence of a certain genetic marker for increased risk of a type of cancer may be reported only as "positive" or "negative." To determine whether the test is a prognostically useful discovery, investigators may follow a group of people, who have been classified as having the marker present or absent, for the rest of their lives. Their death certificates and medical records may then be examined to see whether they ever had the cancer in question. Perhaps some of those with the marker will remain free of the disease, and some of those classified as negative will have the disease. Presumably, the rate of illness is higher among the positives than among the negatives. The issue is whether the difference in the rates is higher than one would expect by chance alone.

Table 3

Proportions of a Population Who Test Positive for a Disease Marker (by Disease Status)

	Disease status		
	+	−	Total
Marker status			
+	a	b	a + b
−	c	d	c + d
Total	a + c	b + d	a + b + c + d

In Table 3, *a* denotes the number of people who are positive for both the marker and the disease, *b* denotes the number of people who are positive for the marker but don't have the disease, *c* indicates the number who are negative for the marker and have the disease, and *d* indicates the number who are negative for both the marker and the disease. The total number of people under study is $a + b + c + d$. What the investigators hope for is the ideal situation in which everyone in the study is in either box *a* or box *d*. Nonzero values for *b, c,* or both indicate imperfection in the test; the greater the number of people in boxes *b* and *c,* the worse the test.

In fact, two extremes are possible: everyone could be in box *a* or

d, and no one in box b or c, meaning that there is a perfect association between the marker and the illness, or there could be no association whatsoever between the marker and the illness. In the latter
case, the proportion of persons with the disease among the marker-
positive persons would be the same as the proportion of persons with
the disease among the marker-negative people. Likewise, the proportions of disease-free people in the marker-positive and -negative
groups would be identical. That is, *a* / *a* + *b* would be the same as *c* /
c + *d*, and *b* / *a* + *b* would be the same as *d* / *c* + *d*. It shouldn't be in-
ferred that being marker positive and being marker negative are
equally likely, or that having the disease and being disease free are
equally likely. When there is no association, it simply means that
whatever proportion of a particular variable is found, that proportion prevails within each category of the other variable.

What usually happens in practice is that observed data follow a pattern between these two extremes, being neither perfectly associated
nor perfectly unassociated. Even a true biological association may not
show up as perfect, because of chance factors; even when there is no
biological association, chance fluctuation may result in proportions
varying slightly (or even greatly) from those expected. The question
is whether the supposed association shown in a table of data repre-
sents more than chance. We need a *P* value that answers the question,
"If two variables in fact were unassociated, what is the probability
that we would see proportions varying to this degree?" In other
words, we need to know how surprising it is that we would find, by
chance alone, such a concentration of people in boxes *a* and *d* and
such a dearth of people in boxes *b* and *c*.

The mathematics of such calculations have been thoroughly
worked out, based on a distribution called the *chi-square distribution,*
and a test called the *chi-square test* is a common test for determining whether there is an association between categorical variables. In
performing this test, you must calculate expected values for each box
(or "cell"), such as *a, b, c,* and *d*. These are the expected values for each

cell under the null hypothesis. If the null hypothesis is true, the same proportions of diseased and nondiseased persons are to be found within each marker status. Values such as those listed as totals in Table 3 are called *marginal totals*, and they are used to obtain these proportions. In Table 3, the overall proportion of people with disease is $(a + c) / (a + b + c + d)$. The overall proportion of people free of disease is $(b + d) / (a + b + c + d)$. Whatever these proportions come out to be, they are multiplied by the total number of marker-positive persons $(a + b)$ to obtain the expected numbers that should be in boxes a and b, if there is no association. Similarly, the proportions are multiplied by the total number of marker-negative persons $(c + d)$ to obtain the expected numbers for boxes c and d.

By collecting actual data, we obtain observed numbers for a, b, c, and d. The sum of the differences between the observed and expected values for each of the boxes in the table is a key element in the calculation of the chi-square value for that table. The differences for each box are then squared, so that the positive and negative differences do not cancel each other out, and they are finally divided by the expected values for each box so that the size of the numbers of observations may be taken into account. After all, a deviation of 3 people from the expected value in a cell means more when the whole sample is 40 than when it is 4,000. This calculation process yields the chi-square statistic. Tables of chi-square values are available in books and computer programs, with P values provided for various levels of this statistic. The smaller the P value for a set of observed data, the less likely that the observed association has occurred by chance alone as a random pile-up into particular cells.

The published P values for the chi-square distribution become less valid as sample sizes decrease. It is a well-known mathematical property of chi-square calculations that the calculation process does not adequately account for the large sampling fluctuations that may be found by chance alone when the sample size is small. At modest sample sizes, you can use what is known as *Yates's correction*, which you probably encounter occasionally in the medical literature. The correction involves the subtraction of a small amount from the chi-square value, making it a bit more difficult to prove significance. This is said to make the test "more conservative" and offsets the ease with which one or two people in a particular category can make a set of observed tabular data show a significant association when sample sizes are small.

However, there is a point at which even this correction fails to deal adequately with the problem, a point at which the sample is too small to permit the use of chi-square, corrected or uncorrected, because the approximation provided by the adjusted distribution is incapable of giving a *P* value that correctly incorporates the sampling variability in tables based on very small numbers. When is it no longer valid to use chi-square? There is some controversy among statisticians about this matter, because the decision whether an approximation is close enough for use is subjective. However, a rule often followed is that if the expected value in any cell of a 2×2 table is less than 5, recourse should be had to *Fisher's exact test*, and chi-square should not be used.

Fisher's is an exact test in the sense that it's the result of calculations that directly give the specific probabilities of each possible way that a given number of people can end up distributed among the cells of a 2×2 table. It is an exact and direct calculation in the same sense that it would be exact and direct to calculate the probability that I'd get one, two, three, four, or five heads when tossing a coin five times, using the binomial distribution. Similarly, with Fisher's exact test, one does not calculate a statistic such as chi-square or *t* and then look up the corresponding *P* value in a table. Consequently, the usual procedure is to enter four values on the computer for the four observed cells of the table and get the probability of the observations. Once again, the calculation is performed under the null hypothesis that there is no association between the two variables.

Notice that not all variables that we might be interested in have only two categories. Stage of disease, for example, usually has more than two categories, and choice of treatment regimen may, also (for example, chemotherapy, radiation, chemotherapy plus radiation, or surgery). The procedure described earlier for the calculation of chi-square statistics is also followed when variables possess more than two categories. However, when P values are calculated for the likelihood of observed tables of data, the number of categories in the table must be taken into account. The published tables of chi-square statistics and their P values are keyed to data tables' category dimensions through the use of something called *degrees of freedom* (or *df*).

Degrees of freedom are calculated as (number of rows − 1) (number of columns − 1). This product tells you how many pieces of information you have in a data table as a consequence of the number of categories. For example, Table 3 is a "2 × 2 table," since it has two rows and two columns; you can calculate that it has one degree of freedom. Suppose you have the table filled out as consisting entirely of expected values. Now you substitute the observed data values in cells a, b, c, and d. How much information is contained in the table of data compared to the null hypothesis table of expected values? You can really consider the data as adding only one piece of information: put an observed value in any one of the four cells, and the numbers for the other three cells can be obtained by subtraction, using the one initial observed value that you supply and the preexisting marginal totals. The differences between your observed data and the expected value table could be generated by any one of the pieces of data. Once you have one cell, the other three cells are not free to vary. This is what is meant by saying that a 2 × 2 table has one degree of freedom. One could imagine other ways of keying P values for chi-square statistics to the number of table categories, but this method is used because it is used in the mathematical derivation of the probabilities associated with various chi-square values.

Not only the number of categories, but also the number of variables can exceed two. Any number of variables may be used in what is called *multidimensional contingency table analysis.* For example, you may be interested in knowing whether there is an association between obstetrical delivery method (caesarean vs. vaginal), ethnic group (for simplicity's sake let's assume two categories, but this is not a requirement for analysis), and the presence or absence of a certain problem in newborns. This is a three-dimensional table that could be represented in two ways. You could make two tables like Table 3, one showing delivery method and ethnic group for newborns with the problem and the other showing delivery method and ethnic group for newborns without the problem. Or you could make a cube table coming out of the paper, with $2 \times 2 \times 2$ categories. The cube is the better way, because it more accurately reflects what actually happens when such a table is analyzed: the data are all considered simultaneously in a three-way calculation of chi-square that helps determine whether there are any associations among the variables.

Higher-dimension tables are more difficult (or impossible) to visualize. I've published a multidimensional contingency table analysis with 10 variables, without being able to picture what is referred to mathematically as a "10-dimensional hyperspace." However, the mathematical treatment of these complex tables is not particularly problematic; it's the same whether 3 or 30 variables are used. *P* values can be calculated to see whether certain variables are associated with the distribution of others. Sometimes a variable has an effect only if another variable is present or absent, that is, only when people are in a particular category (or categories) as far as a different variable is concerned. This situation is termed an *interaction,* and the variable is said to have a *synergistic effect* with another.

Many interesting and complex questions can be addressed by multidimensional contingency table analysis, but the calculations of *P* values cannot be done by hand or even explained in a book of this nature. Moreover, there are various choices of calculation method, each with its own properties and justifications. Finally, there are limits to this approach to analysis: if you're working with many variables and two or more categories of each variable, you may find that in a particular combination of variables' categories there are only a handful of individuals, providing meager statistical power. Thus a very sophisticated analysis may not be warranted.

Regression

Medical researchers are often interested in estimating an equation that describes the relationship between two variables and commonly use *regression* methods for this purpose. Two such variables might be drug dose and some physiological response as an outcome measure. Here the drug dose to which patients are randomized is called the *independent variable*, and the physiological response to that dose is called the *dependent variable*. Conceptually, each patient provides a point on a graph, a point whose coordinate on the x-axis (the horizontal axis) is the dose and whose coordinate on the y-axis is his or her measured outcome. Then a best-fitting line is drawn among the points. This line, called the *least squares line*, is the best-fitting line by a specific mathematical criterion, as follows. For a line drawn through the points, you could measure the up-and-down distance from the line to each and every point on the graph and sum these differences (distances). Such sums would vary among the possible lines you could draw. The line that has the smallest sum of the differences fits best. Actually, some of the differences are positive (upward) and some are negative (downward), and the best-fitting line imaginable would fit exactly through the middle of the cloud of points, dividing it exactly in two, so the sum of differences would be zero. Thus the sum is not used directly, but rather the differences are squared first to get rid of the negative signs, and so the criterion is the minimum sum of *squares* of deviations from the line; hence the name *least squares line*.

There is an equation to every straight line in a plane. In statistics, it's conventional to say that the equation for the least squares line that has been fitted to data is a *model* of the relationship between the two

___

variables *x* and *y*. It is also conventional to say that *x predicts y* according to the equation, since a value for *x* can be put into the equation, and after some arithmetic the corresponding value of *y* can be obtained. What is obtained as a predicted value of *y* is the mean value, according to the model, for all people at dose value *x*. This is your best single estimate of a *y* value. Of course, at dose *x*, there will be a spread around that average *y* value, as a result of person-to-person variability among those at dose *x*. In regression in particular, this random variability is called *error*.

Of course, the procedure of plugging in *x* and obtaining *y* is more reliable when interpolation is being done than when extrapolation is being done. That is, since the equation has been estimated based on a set of data, it is reasonable to expect that the process of plugging in a specific dose and obtaining an estimate of response will result in a better estimate of response over the range of doses for which data have actually been collected. This is true even when the dose plugged in as an *x* value is intermediate between two doses actually observed. Extrapolation is riskier and involves extending the line out beyond the observed range of *x* that had been used to estimate the equation in the first place. The relationship between *x* and *y* might change drastically outside the observed range of *x*.

In regression analysis, the null hypothesis is that the slope of the line is equal to zero. If there is no effect of dose on the physiological measure being studied, as you go horizontally on the graph from one dose to the other the line will neither rise nor fall, so the slope will be zero. Mathematical methods have been developed that take into account the sample size, the spread of the points, and the slope, and permit the estimation of *P* values. Of interest is whether the slope is different from zero more than it would be by chance. If it is, we say that the relationship between *x* and *y* is statistically significant. This test involves the ratio of the slope to the standard error of the slope, in the signal-to-noise format discussed earlier. The magnitude of the effect is also of interest. That is, it is possible to determine with regression the size of the increase in *y* that is obtained for a given in-

A Regression Line

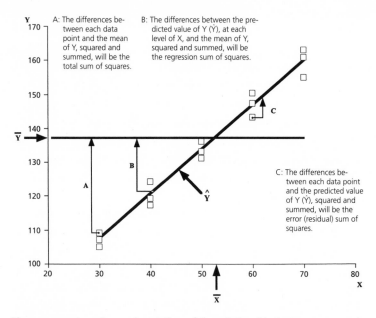

Linear regression gives a description of the relationship between two variables, x and y, in the form of a straight line, and provides the equation for that line. It also lets us test the relationship for statistical significance. Suppose that the figure above shows the relationship in adulthood between age (on the x-axis) and systolic blood pressure (in millimeters of mercury, on the y-axis). We have three observations, represented by boxes, at each 10-year age point. The overall mean age in the whole data set is about 52.5 and is indicated by an arrow pointing to the x-axis ($\overline{X}$); the overall mean value for blood pressure is about 138, and a horizontal line indicates its position on the y-axis ($\overline{Y}$). The diagonal line summarizes the overall relationship between x and y in the data points and, in fact, is a series of estimates of the value of y most likely to be seen at the various ages. The estimates are average values of y for each age x. These estimates are sometimes called *predicted* values of y, and are denoted by the symbol $\hat{Y}$.

The overall mean value of *y* is quite important when we wish to determine whether the regression is statistically significant. This determination requires three key calculations. First, as typified by arrow A in the diagram, the vertical difference from every observed data point to the mean *y* value is obtained, squared, and summed; this is usually referred to as the total *sum of squares*. It's the sum of squared deviations from the mean value. The differences denoted by arrow B are taken next. These are the vertical differences from the *predicted* values to the mean *y* value. Squaring and summing them gives the *sum of squares due to regression*. You can see that if all the data were to lie precisely on a straight line, the total sum of squares and the sum of squares due to regression would be equal numbers. However, with data from the real world, such perfection is not to be expected. The difference between the sums of squares obtained from real versus predicted values is called *error*, or *residual variability*.

In short, all the variability in the system—that is, all deviation of all observations from the mean value of systolic blood pressure—can be divided up into two pieces. First there is progressive deviation of the regression line from the mean value; then there is deviation of the actual observed points, in turn, away from the regression line. Medical researchers commonly report the first, as a fraction of all variability, and it is this fraction being discussed when you read in the journals about "the proportion of variability explained by regression." Statistical significance is calculated from a ratio: the regression sum of squares to the error or residual sum of squares, with sample size taken into account.

---

crease in *x*. This is determined by the use of the *regression coefficients*, provided by the estimation of the equation. If regression shows that systolic blood pressure (SBP) is obtained by adding 100 to 1.2 times your age, for each increase in age by 1 year, an increase in SBP of 1.2 mmHg occurs, on average. Here 1.2 is the regression coefficient.

Note that this model is appropriate (and gives accurate results for effect sizes, the prediction equation, and P values) only if the relationship between x and y is in fact linear in the range of x under study. A least squares line can be run through many sets of points for which it is inappropriate. If, when graphed, the data have the shape of a rainbow, but tilted up at an angle, a least squares line can be fitted to these points but is really not an accurate description of it. Prediction would not be good, and it might be better to use a curvilinear regression model. Model fitting for curvilinear regression models is more complicated than simple linear least squares fitting, but the interpretation of the output is similar.

The assumptions required for the appropriate use of least squares linear regression may be summarized in the acronym *LINE*. L refers to the assumed linearity of the data, a property that we have just discussed. I stands for independence: the observations are assumed to be independent of one another. N stands for normality. For each value of x, the values of y should be normally distributed. This means that the regression line, as it passes over each value of x on the x-axis, should pass right through the center of those y values that are scattered up and down, above that value of x. In fact, that central y value through which the prediction line passes should be the mean value for y that we would find for that value of x. This mean value corresponds to the predicted value, and the predicted value should, after all, be our most reasonable expectation of what we should see in terms of the y observed for a given value of x. The best guess of what we'd find for y at a given value of x is the average value, and more and more extreme values of y found at that x should be rarer and rarer. Thus, a regression line possesses the properties we expect of it, as long as it has been calculated for data that meet the assumption of normality for values of y at each x value. Finally, E stands for equality of variances. The amount of variability in y must not vary much from x value to x value, if the P values are to be valid. Equality of variability is sometimes called *homoscedasticity* (as opposed to heteroscedasticity).

More than one variable may affect the dependent variable, and regression methods have been developed to allow the estimation of *multiple regression* models. These models allow the estimation of the independent and unique contribution of each of several variables to an overall equation model predicting the outcome variable. For all variables in the model, the magnitude of their effects can be tested for significance and compared. For example, body weight, age, and dose might all have an effect on blood pressure. If all three are in the model at the same time, we get estimates of the contribution of each to blood pressure. Perhaps dose lowers blood pressure, and weight and age raise it, but if they're in the model together, the magnitude of the effect of each is measured and tested for significance separately. Measurement here means that an estimate is obtained for the coefficient for each variable. You may have read in the literature of *forward stepwise regression,* in which models are sequentially estimated as variables are added in order of their importance. At a certain point, when the addition of more of the variables does not significantly improve the overall fit of the model, an optimal model has been obtained. Alternatively, in *stepdown* or *backwards stepwise regression,* a model with lots of variables is sequentially pared down so that it includes only the most significant ones. In regression with more than one variable, each variable must satisfy the assumptions summarized in LINE.

Sometimes in regression analysis the dependent outcome is in essence a yes/no variable, that is, a binary variable having two classifications. For example, during an outbreak of a food-borne disease, a group of people who attended a certain luncheon might be studied. The amounts of various foods and drinks consumed by each individual might constitute a set of independent variables. The dependent variable might be the answer to a yes/no question: whether or not the individual was one of the luncheon attendees who ended up with a lab-confirmed diagnosis of salmonella. *Logistic regression* is used to determine the effects of variables on the probability of the food poisoning occurring (or not). In logistic regression, as in linear regression, the coefficients are tested for significance and the magnitude of the effects is obtained from them. The magnitude of the effects here is measured in terms of the increase in the probability of the dependent variable occurring given unit increases in the independent variables. Stepwise procedures are commonly used in multiple logistic regression, as they are in multiple linear regression.

Correlation

Sometimes in medical research what's needed is not a prediction but a measure of association. For example, in obstetrics, the size of a certain fetal bone, determined by ultrasonography, may be useful as a measure of fetal age. In general, as one variable increases, the other increases, so we say that there is a *correlation*, in this case a positive correlation. A correlation can also be negative of course, meaning that as one increases, the other decreases in an inverse association. The two main questions we're interested in are, Is the association beyond what one might expect by chance? If it is, how "tight," or perfect, is this association?

These questions are answered by calculating P values based on a bivariate normal distribution. That is, we assume both variables to be normally distributed: each observation in the sample consists jointly of one value from one of the normal distributions and the corresponding value from the other distribution. The mathematics of the situation permits the calculation of the probability of obtaining a particular set of such pairs of corresponding values. The summary statistic relating the observations to the P values is called the *correlation coefficient,* or r. Values of r range from -1.00 (perfect negative association) to $+1.00$ (perfect positive association). An association of zero means that knowledge of x has absolutely no predictive value with respect to whether the value of y will be high or low. With an r of zero, a graph of x versus y would look like a handful of buckshot thrown onto a piece of paper: a bunch of dots with no upward or downward tilt. The opposite extreme, a perfect association, is rare in nature; an r of $+1.00$ or -1.00 implies that it is invariably the case that the two variables increase (or decrease) in tandem. An example of a perfect correlation is the association between weight in grams and weight in ounces, but it is difficult to think of a situation in biology where a truly perfect association does not arise from some artifact of measurement such as this.

The square of the correlation coefficient, or r^2, can be shown mathematically to represent the proportion of variability "explained" by the correlation. That is, r^2 answers the question, "What proportion of the variability in x is explained by its association with y?" In another refinement of correlation analysis, a *multivariate* correlation coefficient, or R, can be calculated, based on multivariate normal distributions, by extension and analogy to the bivariate normal distribution. If every variable that has an impact on a variable were known and measured, the proportion of variability explained would be 1.00, and if you knew the value of all but one of the variables, the last value would be completely determinate. It is important to mention that the correlation coefficients discussed so far measure the degree of linear correlation; if all the observations were to lie exactly on a wavy line, the linear correlation coefficient would certainly not be 1.00, but there would be a high degree of association between values on the two variables. Finally, there is a nonparametric linear correlation coefficient that is analogous to the linear correlation coefficient and is calculated from the jointly ranked observations.

A word of caution is in order. Correlation does not imply causality. Correlation may or may not be explained by the influence of one of the factors on the other. For example, a fracture index derived from the number and severity of fractures would be closely correlated with the number of days the patient stays in the hospital, and for good causal reasons. Husbands' weights correlate with wives' weights, for a mixture of causal and noncausal reasons. Perhaps peo-

Correlation Coefficients

If *x* and *y* are unrelated, it means that as one increases there is no particular tendency for the other to increase. In such a circumstance, a graph of the data may look like panel A (right), and the correlation coefficient, *r*, is zero. Panels B and C show data with correlation coefficients of 0.5 and 0.9, respectively. As the correlation coefficient increases, the relationship becomes tighter. (A negative sign in front of the correlation coefficient would indicate that the oval swarm of points turns downward, rather than upward, as you go from left to right across the graph.)

It's extremely important to remember that correlation coefficients measure the degree of *linear* association. If the data are not linear, the correlation coefficients are misleading. For example, in panel D, *r* is calculated to be zero, but there's a distinct curvilinear pattern in the data, as one might find with some dose-response curves in pharmacology. Thus the use of *r* to describe this relationship is inappropriate. In panel E, another distinct curvilinear pattern is seen. Even though *r* is calculated to be nonzero and is rather substantial at 0.5, its use should be avoided here, too; it's not an appropriate descriptor for this nonlinear data set.

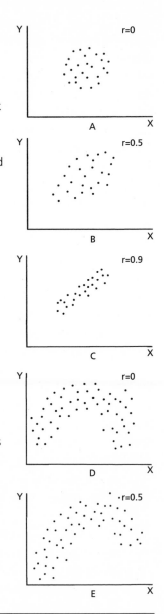

ple are a bit more likely to marry someone similar in size to themselves than to marry someone of quite different size, but husbands and wives also may have more dietary factors in common than two randomly selected people. Finally, a presumably noncausal, or at least not directly causal, correlation may be observed if one examines each year's statistics over the course of American history: there is a strong positive correlation between the number of Presbyterian ministers in the United States and sales of whiskey. This has not occurred because the ministers are making, selling, or drinking the whiskey, or driving their flocks to drink. As the United States has grown, so has the numbers of ministers, and so has liquor consumption. So beware when you see a correlation between any two variables. The correlation may be quite real but noncausal, owing its existence to the fact that some other factor influences both of the variables under study, while they remain quite unaffected by each other.

Hazards Models: Kaplan-Meier Curves and the Cox Model

In medicine, risks (or hazards) are important subjects of study. Examples include the frequency of side effects of a new medication and the comparative mortality of patients with a certain cancer, with and without radiation treatment. Alternatively, the risks, or probabilities of occurrence, may pertain to something we want to happen: we may examine the chance of getting pregnant, for example, and compare the probabilities of doing so among patients in a fertility clinic who are undergoing various treatments.

A key element in the analysis of risks is time. Risks are measured for a specified unit of time, and statements of risk are meaningless without this time specification. After all, what is the probability of mortality if time is not specified? It's 1.0 if the probability of lifetime mortality is meant, and it's practically zero if mortality in the next moment is meant. In cancer research, 5-year survival rates are commonly used. This measure is defined as 1 − the probability of being dead 5 years after diagnosis or after the start of some treatment. This is a handy summary measure, but it doesn't provide information about the shape of the survivorship curve, information that would be given by a graph with time on the x-axis and "proportion still surviving" on the y-axis. The shape of the survivorship curve may have important implications for your patients! For example, a comparative study of patients receiving two different chemotherapeutic agents may show that the 5-year survival rates are identical in the two groups: each is 60%. However, if all the mortality in treatment group A occurs the day after initiation of treatment, and all the mortality in treatment group B occurs one day short of the 5-year measurement point, you want your patients on treatment B.

In general, it may be important to follow up the group(s) under study for a long period of time. Ideally, the group should be followed until every patient in the group has died or experienced the study outcome (for example, pregnancy). Only then do you have the full ability to compare how the treatments affected mortality or another outcome. In practice, of course, there are very real limitations to how long a study can continue. But it must be remembered that, just as with regression lines, the observed experience permits conclusions only about experience in the observed range of x, that is, the observed range of durations from the start of the study. There are many examples of treatments that provide substantial improvement in mortality risk in the short term, with longer follow-up showing that the protective effect diminishes, leaving patients as badly off as untreated patients or even worse off. Even if this cross-over effect is not present, very long term studies of the risks, benefits, and costs are essential for some chronic conditions. For example, the risk of reinfarction after an initial myocardial infarction (MI) and the risk of MI in patients who have had coronary artery bypass grafts can be studied usefully only in the long term. Finally, in a condition of long duration, such as HIV infection, a change in the mortality risks over a long duration of therapy is what is important in some studies.

Some treatments for infertility have the property that if they're going to work, they work in an initial time period. Beyond that time frame, there is little point to exposing patients to the disadvantages and expense of what is overwhelmingly likely to be an ineffective therapy. It is important to be familiar with this property if it is characteristic of a treatment, and again only a relatively long-term study can elucidate it.

Sometimes the fact that a treatment has varying effects over time is informative. For example, as just mentioned, in the treatment of infertility it is often the case that if a treatment is going to work it does so in the short term; if it does not work in the short term, with each passing month the probability of conception falls back closer to the probability observed among untreated infertile patients. When response to treatment has this characteristic, it is interpreted as indicating heterogeneity in the study population. The population consists of a mixture of those who will and those who will not respond to the therapy, so that those whose problem is solved by the therapy respond right away and there is an ever-smaller proportion of responders in the study group over time. The fact that the therapeutic success rate is at its peak at the start and falls continuously from there tells you that the condition under treatment is caused by a mixture of etiologies, which do not all respond to the treatment in the same way.

Not only is follow-up over time important, and longer follow-up more informative than shorter, but also attention must be paid to obtaining more complete follow-up, that is, gathering long-term follow-up information thoroughly from each patient. In the real world there are study dropouts: people change their minds about participating, or the inconvenience gets to be too much for them, or they move away, or they change health care providers— a whole host of things may interrupt your observation of a particular patient. It is obvious that the more information you have on each patient, the better, because loss of information in effect diminishes your sample size and decreases your statistical power. Statistical power in a follow-up study depends not only on the number of people you have at the outset, but also on how many data points you have on each one. Thus you're better off having information on whether patients are therapeutic successes or failures at the fourth, fifth, sixth month of therapy, and so on. But losses to follow-up are also important because they introduce the possibility of bias. Perhaps the sickest people drop out first, because they cannot bother to go to the medical center or even fill out a postcard and mail it in. On the other hand, perhaps the people who are well block the medical study from their consciousness, go out and play tennis, and never come back. Perhaps the people who have some adverse reaction to the treatment drop out so they don't have to submit to the unpleasant treatment again. If you fail to have information on people for any reason, and the reason for dropping out is at all associated with the probability of treatment success, inaccuracies may be introduced into the estimates of the success rate of the therapy. And in any case, even if a patient's reason for dropping out is unrelated to therapy, it diminishes the sample size, which may spell the difference between the experiment's being informative and uninformative by reducing statistical power.

Although the loss of patients to follow-up is never advantageous, useful information can still be gained from patients whose follow-up is incomplete, through the use of appropriate statistical techniques for the analysis of risks. In a coarse summary measure such as a 5-year survival rate, if a patient is lost to follow-up before the completion of 5 years of observation, his or her data cannot be used at all and do not enter into the calculation. This is a risky way to proceed, wasting time, money, and effort if the patient drops out.

The Kaplan-Meier method gets around this problem, allowing you to use whatever information you have available for each patient. Data are used from the point at which observation began to the last point in time for which there is information on that patient. Patients who drop out or are lost to follow-up for whatever reason are referred to as *censored*, meaning that you don't get to look at their data after a certain period of observation, but you still can use the information on censored patients which was obtained prior to censoring.

In the construction of a Kaplan-Meier curve, time is on the *x*-axis, and the proportion of patients still unaffected by the hazard under study (say, mortality) is usually the variable on the *y*-axis. A patient who dies while under study observation contributes to the rate of survivorship until his or her death. Until that point, the line showing the "proportion remaining well" takes no downward step attributable to that individual. When the individual dies, the curve steps downward. After that point, the person who died is of course removed from both the numerator and the denominator in the calculation of mortality risk.

A censored individual is also removed from both the numerator and the denominator in calculating mortality risks, but this removal occurs at the time point at which censoring takes place. Thus, censored individuals contribute their experience to the accurate estimates of "proportion remaining well" while they're still in the study and information is collected on them. The person-years of exposure to risk during which they remained well are an informative part of the picture of the characteristic curve of early mortality in the condition under study, and that information isn't thrown away. At the same time, there is never a downward step in the survivorship curve due to their (never-observed) mortality. Deaths that occur after an individual has been censored occur among a now smaller group of patients remaining in the study. The mortality rates are computed with the censored person absent from the denominator of the total number of patients, and the person vanishes from view without ever having appeared in the numerator of the death rate.

Sometimes instead of letting the curve turn downward at each instance of mortality, survival data are only available in the form of data tabulated in fixed intervals such as a week, month, or year, perhaps because patient's visits occur at fixed intervals. This is called an *actuarial life table method.* A certain number of people enter each interval by surviving to the start of that interval, such as the second week or the third month of study observation. A certain number do not survive to the start of the next interval. The number of these

A Kaplan-Meier Curve

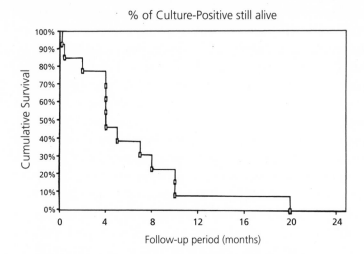

% of Culture-Positive still alive

This figure presents data in the form of a Kaplan-Meier curve. The data concern the mortality experience of a cohort of 20 pediatric AIDS patients who had positive cultures for nontuberculous mycobacteria. Thirteen of the children were known to have died within the 2 years of the study; the 13 boxes marking their durations of survival indicate this. The survival times of the remaining 7 children were unobservable, or "censored": either they were lost to follow-up, or for some other reason data couldn't be obtained from them for the full 2-year period. Thus, there are no boxes to represent them on the graph. However, each of these 7 made a contribution to the proportion surviving throughout the graph up until the point at which he or she was censored. Presenting the entire curve is much more informative than presenting merely median survival time, and since some observations have been censored, the mean survival time cannot be known at all. When two Kaplan-Meier curves are calculated, for example, for two treatment groups, the statistical comparison of the two groups includes the experience represented by the entirety of the two curves.

Source: This figure was originally published in L. Hoyt, J. Oleske, B. Holland, and E. Connor, "Non tuberculous mycobacteria in children with AIDS," *The Pediatric Infectious Disease Journal 11*, (1992): 357, and is reproduced by permission of the Williams & Wilkins Company.

deaths divided by the person-years (person-months, etc.) lived in the interval gives an estimate of the death rate. Patients who are censored are considered to contribute, on average, half of the width of the fixed interval, in terms of personal exposure to risk, but, as in the Kaplan-Meier curve, they're not included in the numerator of the death rate. Both the Kaplan-Meier method and the actuarial life table method make it easy to calculate the median survival time, an important summary comparison measure of mortality; the measure is obtainable as long as the cohort has been followed long enough and with modest losses to follow-up, so that 50% of the original groups have suffered the hazard, such as mortality, that is under study.

If two treatment groups are of interest, you would calculate the downward curves of attrition due to mortality separately for each group but plot them together on the same graph for comparison. In the absence of an association between treatment and the mortality curve, you would find as the result of random fluctuation over the course of observation that sometimes one group's line would be on top, indicating better survivorship, and sometimes the other group's line would be on top. Knowledge of a patient's treatment group would not give a better than 50-50 chance of predicting whether his or her survivorship curve would show better or worse survival than the other curve at a specified duration, and knowing that this patient's group was doing better at one particular duration would tell you nothing about its relative position at the next duration. The other extreme from this "interspersed" situation would be a perfect association between treatment and mortality. The two curves would be entirely disparate, never crossing and never even touching, except at the starting point (time 0), when both groups had 100% of their original numbers.

It's rare to find either of these two extremes of survival curve comparisons. Usually the two curves have a bit, or perhaps a lot, of overlap. How can we decide whether the curves show a difference in principle or whether the differences and overlaps are reasonable to

Statistical Power for Difference in Median Survival Time

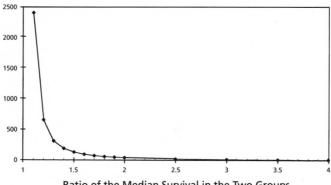

Ratio of the Median Survival in the Two Groups

The graph above shows the sample size a researcher would need to have a 95% chance of having an experiment that is adequate to detect improved survival in the comparison of two treatments that do in fact differ in median survival. With these sample sizes, statistical power is said to be 0.95, since there'll be a 0.95 chance that the results will correctly be declared to be statistically significant; there'll be only a 0.05 chance that because of an unusual sample the two treatment groups will have median values close together and be statistically indistinguishable. The true difference in survival times is measured as the ratio of the median survival times, so a doubling of the median is referred to as "2" on the x-axis, regardless of whether it refers to an improvement from 1 to 2 years or from 1 to 2 decades. We're assuming that the investigator tests with $\alpha = 0.05$ and has complete information on all survival times, with no subjects lost to follow-up or censored in any way. The cumulative decrement in proportions surviving is assumed to be exponential, which is the same as saying that the risks of mortality within each group are constant over time. Such an assumption is common with most tests used to examine the difference between Kaplan-Meier curves.

The point to notice here is the relationship between the size of the difference and the ease with which it's detected. The relationship between these two is not at all linear. If one treatment confers only a doubling, rather than a quadrupling, of median survival, there's not much difference in the sample size required to detect the treatment effect. But to have a successful experiment—that is, to distinguish between an actual difference in survival and a sampling fluctuation—becomes more difficult the smaller the difference in survival is. If a researcher wants to detect a 50% improvement in median survival (that is, a ratio of 1.5), the sample size requirement is less than three times what it is to detect a doubling (ratio of 2.0). However, an improvement measured by a ratio of 1.2 requires a sample five times as large as the sample needed for an improvement measured by a ratio of 1.5. It's mathematically complicated to calculate the function represented by this curve for this rather simple situation; it's even more complicated when there's loss to follow-up and censoring of various kinds; when mortality risks within the groups change over time; or when accrual takes place over an extended period, perhaps differentially by treatment group. Fortunately, computer software exists that allows useful rough calculations of the sample sizes required for a variety of such situations.

---

expect as the result of chance fluctuation? Statistical methods exist that permit the calculation of *P* values for comparisons of Kaplan-Meier curves, and for comparisons of actuarial survival curves. The null hypothesis is that there is no difference between the two curves; the alternative, that they differ more than by chance. The *P* value quantifies the probability that the separations and overlaps between two curves would be observed as a chance fluctuation.

For tests of hypotheses on data presented as Kaplan-Meier curves, one commonly sees in the literature such statistics as Wilcoxon's test, Gehan's test, or Peto and Peto's test; in actuarial work with fixed intervals, one commonly sees reference to the Mantel-Haenszel chi-square test. No one test is best in every situation; the tests differ in various refinements, such as weighting. Weighting is necessary because the probabilities of survivorship at longer durations of observation are determined on the basis of smaller numbers of individuals than those toward the start of the study. So the probabilities of mortality later in the study are not determined with the same degree of certainty as those earlier in the study, since there is more random variation in estimating the probability of mortality with a small sample than there is with a large one. Statisticians have paid much attention to refinements such as these and to the fact that the power to detect the difference between survivorship curves may differ from test to test, depending on the true underlying pattern of attrition, or the differences in levels of mortality that are hypothesized: is it a linear decrease? Is it exponentially declining survivorship? The technical detail of these questions may not be familiar to the clinician, who leaves the choice of test to the biostatistician, but the basic principle is clear: we need an accurate calculation of the probability of seeing this difference between curves if a set of underlying assumptions were true. If the probability is extremely small, the null hypothesis, such as equality of hazards, is considered falsified.

We have seen that in linear regression more than one predictive variable may be of interest. When we are determining influences on survivorship, it may again be of interest to assess the independent and separate impacts of several variables. The hazards model methods and tests just discussed are for use when there is one variable, such as treatment, that is of interest. There may be other variables to consider, for example, age, race, sex, stage of disease, or concomitant illnesses or treatments, which are called *covariates*. It may be possible to produce Kaplan-Meier curves for each category of covariate and determine whether the difference in survivorship owing to treatment occurs within groups defined by membership in the covariate categories. Often sample size precludes this, inasmuch as there aren't enough patients with particular combinations of the covariates to enable us to make curves for each combination. Also, it is not possible in such a framework to compare the magnitude and test the significance of the covariates simultaneously. A final problem is that it is difficult to interpret dozens of pages of curves and tests, comparing the treatments within many categories of covariates.

In this circumstance, the *Cox model,* or *proportional hazards regression,* is useful. The dependent variable is, in essence, the probability of mortality, with all points on the curve considered simultaneously and weighted by sample size and with censoring properly taken into account. As in multivariate regression, one can consider many variables simultaneously and gain from their estimated coefficients a measure of their impact in terms of the increased odds of mortality for each increase in each independent variable. The statistical significance of each variable may be considered, and the impact of each is measured with the others already in the model and implicitly controlled for. The hazards are assumed to be constant within various categories, so if one category is half as risky as another, that ratio of risk is constantly in that proportion throughout the observed period; hence the name *proportional hazards regression.* However, there are some ways of getting around this limitation if the hazards are not believed to be in constant proportions, such as a method allowing the inclusion of variables that represent the unique effect of being in a particular time interval. Analysis of the probability structure of the whole model results in the calculation of *P* values, which have the same interpretation as always: under a null hypothesis that this variable has no effect, is the concentration of mortality in a particular category or categories something that is very surprising by chance alone? If it is, a statistically significant determinant of mortality has been identified by analyzing the data according to this model.

Confidence Intervals

The results of medical research are increasingly presented in terms of *confidence intervals* in addition to or instead of *P* values. The basic principle is the same in both statistical approaches: a null hypothesis is of interest, and a set of observations is compared with what would be expected based on that hypothesis and probability mathematics.

Let's pick a simple case for an example. Say we have the mean of an observation from a single sample. The data that are being averaged are the weight changes in kilograms in a group of people on a weight loss regimen. A reasonable null hypothesis might be that the average individual on the weight loss regimen has a value of zero for the weight change variable. Here we use our sample mean as an estimate of the true mean change in a population on this regimen. Instead of using probability mathematics to assess the chance of seeing such a sample (as is done for *P* values), we use it to construct an upper bound and a lower bound around the mean change. These are called the *upper and lower bounds of the confidence interval.* A confidence interval is constructed for some quantified level of confidence; 95% and 99% confidence intervals are usually used.

Calculation of a 95% confidence interval produces a range of possible values for the true mean (the mean for the whole population). We can be 95% certain that the true mean falls somewhere in this range, which was calculated using the sample mean value, the sample size, and a bit of probability mathematics. A 99% confidence interval is always a wider range of values than a 95% confidence interval, because if you want more certainty that your range of values includes the true one, you have to include more values. After all, if you wanted 100% certainty you'd have to include an infinite range of values. Also, as the sample size goes up, the confidence interval gets narrower and narrower, because the sample mean becomes a better and better estimator of the population mean. If you had the entire population as your sample, the sample mean would be the population mean, and the confidence interval would be not an interval, but a point.

Practically speaking, we can never be perfectly certain about the conclusions we make about a population on the basis of a sample from it, whether the values we examine are *P* values or confidence intervals. All we can do is to quantify sampling error. A confidence interval has the specified probability of containing the mean of the population from which the sample was drawn, as long as we sample from a distribution and do the arithmetic needed to construct the interval from the sample. Thus, 95% of possible samples will have means such that the confidence interval based on them will contain the true population mean. But then it follows that 5% of such intervals will *not* contain the true population mean, so there is a 5% chance of being wrong with respect to the location of the true mean. Five percent of the time you will have a sample so far away from the true mean of the population that a confidence interval based on it does not extend to include the true mean. Earlier, we discussed why an alpha level of 0.05 means we have a 5 percent chance of being wrong and erroneously declaring a difference to be significant. Similarly, a 95% confidence interval around a mean might include all positive numbers or all negative numbers, thus excluding a value of zero. The conclusion, offered with 95% certainty, would then be that the mean change is not zero, so that the hypothesis of no change is not supported. This is the same thing as saying the *P* value of this set of observations under the null hypothesis is 0.05. Indeed, the arithmetic of *P* values and confidence intervals makes them consistent statistics when performed on a given sample. A sample that causes you to consider the null hypothesis not supported by the evidence at $\alpha = 0.05$ (two-tailed) will also result in a 95% confidence interval that does not bracket the mean value required by the null hypothesis. Confidence intervals are ordinarily two-tailed, except when this would lead to impossible values, such as negative mortality rates.

Some researchers prefer confidence intervals over *P* values because they provide a range of values, rather than a yes/no decision criterion. They figure that the reader is freer to draw his or her own conclusions after examining the confidence interval and seeing how

Confidence Intervals

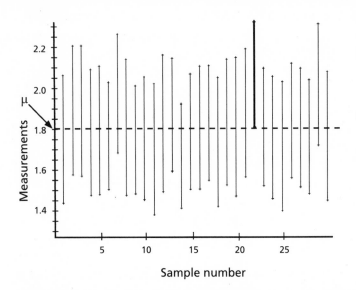

Sample number

Although a confidence interval is constructed from the data in hand from a single sample, its key property is perhaps best understood by considering the confidence intervals constructed on the basis of lots of samples. Suppose we've been drawing samples, each having 20 observations, from a very large population with a mean physiological measurement value (μ) of 1.802. So far, we have 30 such samples drawn, and from each we've calculated a 95% confidence interval. The diagram above shows the results.

For convenience, the dotted line indicates the constant true value of 1.802. Each vertical line shows the range of the 95% confidence interval for one of the samples. Recall from the text that confidence intervals around a mean value are symmetrical: the centerpoint of each one of these confidence intervals is the mean value of the sample from which it was calculated.

Suppose we didn't know that the true mean value in the population is 1.802, and we had only one of the samples to go by. This is the usual case in clinical research. We'd have to rely on that sample's mean as an estimate of the population mean. By and large, the confidence intervals are centered on the true population mean, and they almost always include it; but once in a while, as a result of sampling fluctuation, a sample is fairly wide of the mark. When we calculate a 95% confidence interval based on our sample, the key property is that we're 95% certain that the true population mean (in the group from which our sample was drawn) lies between two numbers. These numbers are the upper and lower bounds of our confidence interval. Ninety-five percent of such confidence intervals will in fact contain the true population mean, but 5% will not. Thus, on average, one such confidence interval out of 20 will not include the true population mean, and the investigator will state that the sample mean is statistically distinguishable from μ (in this case 1.802). In our computer trial of 30 samples, one confidence interval based on a sample of 20 did not include the true population mean, as indicated by the bold vertical line representing sample number 22.

---

closely it comes to touching the null value and how much it extends in the two directions. Indeed, it is sometimes of considerable clinical interest to read that a certain mean value may range (with 95% certainty) from as low as x to as high as y. In any case, researchers could considerably improve the presentation of P values from significance tests by reporting actual observed P values, instead of stating simply that a finding was "not significant at $\alpha = 0.01$." It may interest the reader of a journal article to know that a certain finding would be expected by chance 0.02 or 0.05001 of the time, rather than 0.98 of the time.

Although we've concentrated on one particular example, confidence intervals may be constructed around almost any statistical measure of medical importance that is being estimated from a sample. Earlier we described such measures as means and differences in means, proportions and differences in proportions, regression slopes, regression coefficients, mortality curves, and estimates of the effects of variables on mortality curves using the Cox model. All these, and many other statistical measures, can have confidence intervals constructed around them, and many such confidence intervals may be seen in any recent issue of a typical medical journal.

Three

Your Patient Tests Positive

Is Disease Present?

Health care providers often have recourse to clinical lab tests as an aid in diagnosis. Depending on the suspected illness, lab tests may be an important or even a mandatory part of the diagnosis procedure. We tend to accept lab results as important and, sometimes, definitive information and expect that a good clinical lab, adhering rigorously to appropriate procedures, gives accurate results. Remember that there are two measures of the accuracy of the results of a lab test. The first is *precision*, which refers to the reproducibility of the results. If the lab test is precise, results from the same sample should show little variability. A bathroom scale lacks precision if it shows a wildly different value each time its stepped on by the same person in the space of an hour. The second measure is *bias*. If a test is biased, it means that the results, on average, do not center on the true value. We want lab procedures and practices that are unbiased, so that on average there is no deviation from the truth. A bathroom scale that may be precise in terms of yielding exactly the same measurement every time it's stepped on by the same person may nonetheless be biased, always showing a value precisely 10 pounds too low or too high. Ideally, we want an *accurate* scale, one that is both precise and unbiased, although a problem of bias is usually easier to fix, through calibration or rescaling, than is a problem of imprecision. Sometimes, as with some blood cell counts, there is little bias but values fluctuate wildly, not because of ineptitude on the part of the lab, but because the biological measurement is inherently "noisy," or highly variable. In such measures we must accept a lack of precision.

Even if a lab procedure is shown to be highly precise and unbiased, and the lab performing the test does so carefully and without committing any error, a diagnostic result may have a devastatingly low probability of reflecting the patient's true disease status. To what extent can you have faith in a clinical lab test result? The answer depends on the prevalence of the disease in question in the population from which the patient is drawn. The need to consider disease prevalence may surprise the clinician, who is perhaps accustomed to thinking that only the inherent characteristics of the test and the quality of the lab running the test need to be considered in deciding how much credence to give a lab result.

Definitions of the Sensitivity, Specificity, and Predictive Value of Tests

Let's take a moment to define what is meant by the inherent characteristics of a test. The probability that a patient who in fact has the disease gets a correspondingly positive lab result is, let's say, 0.80. This value is represented by $P(T+|D+)$, which is read, "the probability that the test is positive given that the patient is disease positive." This value is called the *sensitivity* of the test. The *specificity* of the test, $P(T-|D-)$, is the probability that a patient who is disease free is correctly classified as disease free by the test result. A test's manufacturer generally estimates the test's sensitivity and specificity before making it commercially available, by obtaining test results among people who have been diagnosed as disease positive and disease negative by some gold standard diagnostic test, such as clinical exam, biopsy, symptoms, radiography, or perhaps a combination of these.

These inherent sensitivity and specificity values, although important measures of a test's accuracy, are not what you really need to know when you're taking care of patients, however. You need to know $P(D+|T+)$, the probability that the disease is in fact present if the test is positive. After all, the information on the sheet from the lab says that the patient has a positive test result, so *that* is the given piece of information that you need to interpret; what you need to know is how often that piece of lab data is correct. $P(D+|T+)$ is called the *predictive value of the positive test*. The probability that a patient is disease free if the lab report shows a negative test is $P(D-|T-)$, the *predictive value of the negative test*.

Suppose that 5% of a population has a disease. We might say the prevalence is 0.05 and denote it by $P(D+)$. Of course, that would make the proportion of the population without the disease, or $P(D-)$, 0.95. Suppose we're using a test with a sensitivity of 0.80 and a specificity of 0.90. What would be the predictive values of a positive test and a negative test? To answer this question, we construct a 2×2 table that subdivides a group of people into those with and without disease and with and without a positive test result. This could be done for an actual population, but usually it's done for a round number from a hypothetical population. With sensitivity, specificity, and prevalence fixed, the proportion of tests that correctly reflect the patient's disease status is fixed, so it doesn't matter what underlying overall number is used to represent the total population.

Suppose we have 1,000 patients. With a disease prevalence of 5%, every 1,000 people with the disease would be divisible into 50 who have the disease and 950 who are disease free. Among the 50 patients with the disease, 80% would test positive for it, because the sensitivity is 0.80. So 40 of those 50 patients would be correctly classified by the test; they're referred to as *true positives*. By subtraction we can see that there would be 10 *false negatives*. The specificity of 0.90 tells us that among every 950 disease-free individuals, 855 negative tests would result. These are *true negatives*. By subtraction we can see that there would be 95 *false positives*. The results are shown in Table 4.

Sensitivity, Specificity, and Predictive Value of a Test

Sensitivity

Notation: $P(T+|D+)$

Definition: If you were to perform a screening test for a particular disease on a group of people who have the disease, the proportion of people classified as positive for the disease by the test is referred to as the *sensitivity* of the test.

Specificity

Notation: $P(T-|D-)$

Definition: If you were to perform a screening test for a particlar disease on a group of people who do *not* have the disease, the proportion of people classified as negative for the disease by the test is referred to as the *specificity* of the test.

Predictive Value of a Positive Test

Notation: $P(D+|T+)$

Definition: The proportion of people who are classified as positive by the screening test for a particular disease and who in fact have the disease is the predictive value of a positive test; for the clinician, it's the probability that a positive screening test is true. The predictive value of a positive test depends not only on how good the test is, but also on the prevalence of the disease (see the text for further discussion).

Predictive Value of a Negative Test

Notation: $P(D-|T-)$

Definition: The proportion of people who are classified as negative by the screening test for a particular disease and who in fact don't have the disease is the predictive value of a negative test; for the clinician, it's the probability that a negative screening test is correct. The predictive value of a negative test depends not only on how good the test is, but also on the prevalence of the disease (see the text for further discussion).

Disease State and Test Results, Cross-Classified

Disease State

Test result	Has disease	Is disease free	Total
Positive	True positive	False positive	All positive tests
Negative	False negative	True negative	All negative tests
Total	All diseased patients	All disease-free patients	All tests and patients

In the scenario in Table 4, out of 135 positive tests that come back from the lab, 40 will be drawn from people with the disease and 95 will be drawn from people who do not have the disease. Thus the proportion of positive tests that correctly indicate that the patient has the disease is 40/135, or 0.296. This number is the predictive value of the positive test. Even though it is a characteristic of the test that $P(T+|D+)$ is 0.80, when a lab report comes to the physician reading "positive" there is only a 0.296 chance—less than 1 in 3—that the patient in fact has the disease.

Table 4
Sensitivity, Specificity, Prevalence, and Predictive Value

	Disease		
	+	−	Total
Test			
+	40	95	135
−	10	855	865
Total	50	950	1,000

Suppose we leave sensitivity and specificity unchanged and alter the prevalence. The prevalence is now 50%, so out of our 1,000 people, 500 have the disease and 500 don't. Eighty percent, or 400, of the 500 people with the disease are true positives. Ninety percent, or 450, of the 500 disease-free individuals are true negatives. The rest of the numbers are obtained by subtraction, and the completed new table is Table 5.

Table 5
Sensitivity and Specificity with Changed Prevalence
and New Predictive Value

	Disease		
	+	−	Total
Test			
+	400	50	450
−	100	450	550
Total	500	500	1,000

Now 400 out of 450 positive tests come from people with the disease, so the predictive value of the positive test is 400/450, or 0.889. In this scenario, when a positive lab result indicates that the patient has the disease, there is a nearly 90% chance that it's correct. Yet the characteristics of the test itself have remained unchanged, and only the prevalence of the illness in the population to which it applied has been altered.

Prevalence has a marked effect on the predictive value of the test, because if a disease is exceedingly rare, most positive readings will be false positives. As the disease becomes more common in a population, it becomes increasingly likely that any particular positive lab test comes from someone with the disease, as true positives come to predominate among the positive readings. This phenomenon may best be seen in the extreme situations. Suppose everyone in a population has a disease. If this is the case, there is no possibility of a false positive and all positives are true positives. In the absence of lab error, the predictive value of a positive test would be perfect. At the other extreme, imagine a population in which the disease is totally absent, so there is no possibility of a true positive; all positives are false positives, and the lab test is always wrong.

The inverse situation exists for the predictive value of a negative test. In Table 4, $P(D-|T-)$ is 855/865, or 0.988. In Table 5 it is 450/550, or 0.818. As the predictive value of a positive test goes up, the predictive value of a negative test goes down. This is because as the disease becomes more prevalent, there are fewer disease-negative people for whom true-negative tests results may be obtained. At the extremes, everyone has the disease so all negatives are false negatives and $P(D-|T-)$ is zero; or no one has the disease, so all negatives are true negatives and $P(D-|T-)$ is 1.0.

The Influence of Prevalence on Test Results

Although these imagined situations may be far-fetched, the principle operates in all intermediate situations and has importance for public policy. It must be remembered, in this age of concern about HIV infection, that the use of a screening test in a low-prevalence population will produce a rich yield of false positives requiring expensive additional clinical investigation before the disease is ruled out. Some thought should be given to whether the money for such a testing program might be better spent. On the other hand, in groups with high prevalence, the excellent reliability of many lab tests makes screening a practice of great clinical utility.

The inherent characteristics of a lab test may be fixed in advance before the test is approved and in clinical use, but only certain aspects are really fixed by the physical and chemical properties of the procedures employed. Often the cutoff used to determine whether a particular sample is to be called normal or abnormal is arbitrary, even though it becomes part of required standard procedure. Unfortunately, there is a trade-off: selection of a cutoff that yields improved sensitivity must have a cost in terms of decreased specificity. Suppose findings above a certain value for intraocular pressure were initially held to be abnormal and diagnostic for glaucoma. Then it is realized that some individuals with the disease but with lower values are being declared disease free by the test. Thus $P(T+|D+)$ might be improved with a lower cutoff, so that patients with lower values of intraocular pressure would also correctly be considered positive for glaucoma by the test. However, the specificity, $P(T-|D-)$, would decrease with the new lower cutoff, because increasing numbers of patients who are disease free would erroneously be declared to have glaucoma. More and more D− patients would lie above the criterion point as it moved lower and lower, and they would be considered positive by the test.

The clinician must realize that there are many sources of uncertainty surrounding lab tests. Lab procedure must be adhered to, but even perfect compliance with protocol rules out only one source of erroneous judgment based on lab tests. Another source of error is discussed in Chapter 1 in the section on errors that occur in hypothesis testing: the use of normal ranges to judge outcomes from many lab tests results in the multiple testing problem and ensures that "abnormal" results are likely to be found due to chance in any long series of lab tests. But in this chapter we have shown that even if only one test is performed, the clinical significance of an abnormal finding may vary a great deal depending on the prevalence of abnormality in the population from which the patient is drawn. In other words, the clinical significance depends on the probability that the patient has the disease to begin with.

This is a fancy way of saying what every clinician knows: clinical knowledge of the patient is often central to deciding whether to accept or disregard a test result. Sometimes we know the patient, so we suspect a false positive and do further tests to confirm this hunch. You may notice that there's something circular in the reasoning that allows us to use our hunch to reject the finding of a lab test that was performed in order to determine whether or not the hunch is true. Clinical hunches about particular patients may be valuable, and they often have a high (but unquantified) probability of being correct. If a lab result turns out to be in conflict with our expectation, we may not know which has a higher probability of being correct, the test or the hunch. That is when the trap of circular reasoning must be escaped with further confirmatory testing. The probability of obtaining by chance alone a positive result on each of a series of ever more sensitive tests is next to nil. That is why a positive ELISA, Western blot, polymerase chain reaction, and viral culture overrule our clinical expectation that a certain individual is not infected with HIV.

4

Epidemiological Study Designs

Epidemiology is the study of the distribution and determinants of disease frequency. It may be divided into descriptive epidemiology and analytical epidemiology. *Descriptive epidemiology* presents information about the distribution of disease according to various factors, usually summarized as factors pertaining to person, place, and time. The emergence of patterns in the occurrence of disease often leads to testable hypotheses about risk factors and their influence on disease etiology; testing of these hypotheses is called *analytical epidemiology.*

Descriptive Epidemiology

As an example, a descriptive epidemiology of schistosomiasis would include maps of its distinctive geographical distribution in moist tropical climates. It would include mention of the types of people who get the disease: people who live near bodies of water, are poor, and use those bodies of water for washing and bathing and as an open sewer. People who live where irrigation ditches are used for agriculture often have this disease. Moreover, the incidence of this illness changes over time: in a drier area an irrigation ditch may be put in, and the incidence of schistosomiasis may then change from low to high. Drain the ditch, and the incidence of new cases falls.

A descriptive study need not be a worldwide survey. Sometimes a description of one unusual case extends epidemiological knowledge, because it establishes that the disease can occur where it had been thought it could not. A case series may describe several unusual cases. These can be important. The reporting of a few cases of Kaposi's sarcoma in young homosexual males in New York, when it had previously been a disease mostly of the elderly and a few ethnic groups, suggested a new and distinctive risk factor for that cancer— HIV infection.

Analytical Epidemiology

Cross-sectional Studies

Once descriptive epidemiology has suggested hypotheses, how are they tested? Researchers might first attempt a *cross-sectional* study. This is basically a survey and a one-shot deal. The risk factors and prevalence of a disease of interest may be determined systematically at the same point in time. This is a relatively quick and cheap type of study to carry out. For example, the prevalence of coronary heart disease and the level of serum cholesterol in a group of people could be determined at one visit. The statistical significance of differences in rates can be established. The problem is that cross-sectional studies do not establish the temporal sequence necessary for drawing inferences about cause and effect. For example, suppose that persons with pneumococcal pneumonia were surveyed, and all were found to have high titers of antibody to the relevant pneumococcal antigen in the blood. What does this prove? Does it show that infection with pneumococcal pneumonia leaves this detectable marker in the blood? Or does it show that it's possible to come down with pneumococcal pneumonia, despite supposedly protective levels of circulating antibody? When a medical phenomenon is not yet well understood, either direction of causality may be a plausible interpretation of data from a cross-sectional study

There are two other broad types of studies that form the bulk of analytical epidemiological studies. These are the case-control study and the cohort study.

Case-Control Studies

In the case-control study we start out with a group of people diagnosed as having the disease. These are the cases. We also have a comparison group of controls. The question we wish to answer is, Do the two groups differ more than would be expected by chance in terms of their previous exposure to a specific factors that are causal agents? If the exposure is the same (within the bounds of chance fluctuation), we've failed to demonstrate a nonrandom association between exposure and disease.

As usual, the sample size must be clearly set in advance in a case-control study, so that we have a reasonable prospect of finding a statistically significant difference that is of clinical interest and is specified in advance. However, there are several additional methodological issues that we must carefully deal with to ensure the validity of our conclusions. Let's start with the collection of cases. Clear diagnostic criteria must be set to define who will be in the study, and these criteria must be adhered to consistently. Cases should have a single type of illness, not a mix of illnesses, because it is difficult to study causation in a group of cases who have illnesses with different etiologies.

Thus we generally study cases who've been diagnosed as having a single type of lung cancer, for example, oat cell carcinoma of the lung. Cases are identified from such sources as disease registries, hospital records, health insurance plans, and the like. Personal exposure information on cases may be obtained from these data sources or from interviews with the cases or their co-workers, families, or associates.

Controls are also drawn from a variety of sources. They may come from the general population or may be co-workers, friends, or associates of the cases. They may be patients hospitalized at the same hospital as the cases, but with different and unrelated disease. Selection of the controls is extremely important, because they must be similar in general to the population from which the cases are drawn. For example, we wouldn't want to compare cancer cases among urban industrial plant workers with controls drawn from farmers from a totally different rural region. A better comparison would be permitted by using controls who are similar to the patient group on a whole list of factors, such as region of residence, ethnic group, and socioeconomic status, but who have been hospitalized for fractures. Then, if we compare, for example, the smoking rate among patients hospitalized for lung cancer with that among patients hospitalized for fractures, differences in smoking rates between the two patient groups will not be due to that list of other factors. We can then make comparisons without wondering whether, for example, differences in air pollution level between two regions, rather than smoking history, explained why some people got cancer and others didn't.

A potential problem with the use of hospital controls is that the risk factors for their illnesses might be the same as the risk factors for the disease under study. Comparing lung cancer patients with patients hospitalized with bronchitis and emphysema, we might find relatively little difference in antecedent exposure. Selection of controls must be performed with caution.

CONFOUNDING VARIABLES

In principle, we want groups who differ only in case/control status and (because of a causal relationship) prior exposure to a risk factor and don't differ in any other way. Thus a comparison of the prior exposures of cases and controls would be the purest measure possible of the etiological significance of the causal relationship under study, free from the taint of confounding variables. A *confounding variable*, or *confounder*, is a variable that is associated with both the exposure of interest and the disease under study. For example, at one time in certain regions of Malaysia, infant mortality was more common among children who had been breastfed for a long time than among those who had been breastfed only a short time. Does this mean that breastfeeding was a risk factor for infant mortality, or that inadequate supplementary and weaning foods were available to children who were breastfed longer? Neither was the case. It was simply that poorer, rural people were more likely to breastfeed their infants than were people living in urban areas, and the city dwellers were more likely to be middle class and to have access to professional health care. So an association arose: the breastfed infant was more likely to die, but for reasons that had nothing to do with breastfeeding and a lot to do with the socioeconomic conditions of those who were breastfeeding.

ADJUSTING FOR CONFOUNDERS: MATCHING, STRATIFICATION, AND REGRESSION

Confounding variables can be dealt with by *matching*, whereby cases and controls are matched on variables that might be confounders. For example, each rural woman who was of a particular social class and whose child had survived infancy could be matched to an urban dweller of the same class whose child had also survived. The same procedure would be followed for cases where the child had died. Then a comparison of breastfeeding histories might or might not show a difference when we compared all infants who died and those who survived, but any difference would not be due to the confounding effects of the variables on which cases and controls were matched. If cases and controls have been matched on a given variable, it is impossible to assess the impact of that variable on the disease, since both groups have been forced to have presumably identical distributions of the matched variable. Also, matching is administratively complex and expensive, may slow down the study or be impossible to obtain, and in any event must be undertaken at the start of the study. Still, there are big advantages to matching, because not only are the effects of confounders minimized, but statistical power increases because interindividual variability is minimized.

Another way to reduce the problem of confounding variables is *stratification*. Here comparisons of cases and controls are made within strata. *Strata* are groups as homogeneous as possible with respect to some variable that might be a confounder. It's as if the study question were being answered from various different groups of people, because the rates of exposure among cases and controls are calculated separately for each category of the suspected confounder. When the statistics have been performed in such a framework, it's reported in the medical literature as a "stratified analysis."

Finally, *regression techniques* can also be used to allow for the effects of confounders. As we've discussed, in multiple regression (and multiple logistic regression) many independent variables can be put into an equation, permitting the simultaneous estimation of the unique impact of each on the dependent variable. If confounding variables are identified and recorded in a study, they can be put into an equation first. The regression coefficient for the variable of interest, obtained next, will show the unique contribution of the variable we're really interested in, as a determinant of the dependent variable, beyond the impact it has because of its associations with the confounders. Thus estimates of the magnitude and statistical significance of the variables of interest are said to be "adjusted for" the impact of the confounders.

DETERMINATION OF EXPOSURE AND DISEASE STATUS

Errors in either exposure or disease information may prevent the accurate estimation of the magnitude of associations. Usually disease status is well documented in a case-control study, since the study team can verify this variable by whatever means they deem suitable. Exposure information pertains to a time in the past, possibly long ago, or perhaps reflects a complicated and undocumented history of exposure, such as employment history or the fluctuating smoking status of an individual. Moreover, recall errors may be biased. Cases are already known to have a disease, so these patients or their doctors or associates may tend to remember exposure to risk factors in the past. They may be prompted to recollect, "Oh, yes, didn't he work in an industrial plant once?" "Yes, I think perhaps he did work with pesticide residues in that plant," they may say. Alternatively, a lung cancer patient, for example, might feel overwhelmed by the thought that his smoking had a part in the etiology of his illness and may be in denial, saying that his smoking was negligible.

Another source of bias in exposure information is that a high rate of missing data concerning exposure variables may mask different rates of nonresponse— different, that is, with respect to the presence or absence of the exposure factor. Perhaps smokers, irritated at being blamed for their lung cancer, will be the very lung cancer patients who do not fill out the form concerning smoking history. There will be a *selection bias* in the response rates. The remaining lung cancer patients may truthfully say they never smoked, and then there might be no reported difference between the rates of smoking among lung cancer patients and their controls.

It's clearly preferable to use exposure information recorded before diagnosis and to corroborate data from one source with those from another. Incorrect classification of cases and controls with respect to exposure may allow bias to creep into retrospective studies. Differential recall of exposure may exaggerate or minimize association between cause and disease. But it is important to be aware that even random unbiased misclassification errors are a problem: such errors reduce the difference between cases and controls in terms of exposure and may reduce a real difference to a level so low that the study cannot detect it. In terms of the signal-to-noise ratio, the signal becomes weaker and weaker as memory loss occurs over time, until the random noise drowns it out. The problem can be seen best in the most extreme circumstance. For example, suppose all lung cancer cases smoked, and no controls smoked. Any error, even if unbiased, will diminish the starkness of this contrast. For example, if 20% of the lung cancer cases were erroneously reported to be nonsmokers, and 20% of the controls were erroneously reported to be smokers, the contrast between the smoking rates of cases and controls would be diminished, even though the misclassification errors are not even biased.

STATISTICAL MEASURES OF ASSOCIATION: THE ODDS RATIO AND ATTRIBUTABLE RISK

What statistical measures of association do we obtain from case-control studies? You may remember seeing odds ratios reported in the literature. The *odds ratio* is the critical measure for assessing the role of a factor in the etiology of a disease in a retrospective study. It is an estimate of relative risk. Relative risk is the ratio of the disease rate among the exposed to the disease rate among the nonexposed. As is discussed later, it can be obtained directly when one is doing a cohort study, but in a case-control study it can only be estimated by the odds ratio. The odds ratio is a good estimate of the relative risk when the disease under study is a comparatively rare one, as is ordinarily the case.

If an odds ratio of 2.0 is calculated from a case-control study, the interpretation is that the chance that a person would get the disease if he or she had been exposed is twice the chance that the person would get the disease if he or she had not been exposed. There are statistical tests for the odds ratio; the null hypothesis is that the odds ratio is equal to 1.0. Remember, if the disease rates are the same regardless of whether exposure to the risk factor occurs, the odds ratio should be 1.0. Anything in excess of an equality of the disease rates indicates risk associated with exposure, but some of this may be due to chance fluctuation, and thus there's a need for statistical tests to determine whether the excess might be due (or is unlikely to be due) to chance. Of course, a certain exposure that we believe before the study to elevate risk might turn out in fact to be protective; then the odds ratio would be less than 1.0. For example, an odds ratio of 0.5 indicates that a disease is half as likely among individuals exposed to a certain factor than it is among unexposed individuals.

There are also a number of statistical measures of *attributable risk* that may be calculated from case-control studies. These measures indicate how much of the disease rate in the population can be attributed to exposure to the factor in question. Whereas the odds ratio tells us about the etiological significance of a risk factor, attributable risk measures tell us primarily about the public health impact that might be seen if the risk factor were eliminated. For example, if the population attributable risk proportion were 0.15, it would mean that 15% of cases of disease are attributed to the factor under study. Attributable risk is a composite of the power of the risk factor as a causative agent and the prevalence of the risk factor in the population. A risk factor may be an extremely powerful causative agent of disease, but if only a handful of people in one industrial plant are ever exposed to that agent, and the disease is also caused by other weaker but more widespread causative agents, eliminating the powerful risk factor might not have much of an impact on rates of the disease as far as the public health is concerned. On the other hand, an exposure that is responsible for only a modest elevation of risk but is widespread may have a substantial impact on the public health.

Cohort Studies

A *cohort* is a follow-up group with something in common during some time span. In a cohort study, the entire group of people selected as a cohort is free of the disease at the start of the project, but different people in the cohort fall into different exposure categories. They are followed up over time. The exposure groups may differ in disease rates, or there may be no difference in disease rates between exposure groups, in which case we have failed to detect an association between exposure and disease.

There are many types of cohorts. There are birth cohorts, college graduation classes, and marriage cohorts. There are cohorts with an unusual experience that is of epidemiological relevance. Survivors of the atomic bomb at Hiroshima are such a group, and it is of interest to compare the subsequent medical histories of the survivors, clas-

Comparison of Case-Control and Cohort Studies

Case-control studies are generally	Cohort studies are generally
• Conducted with smaller samples	• Conducted with larger samples
• Inexpensive	• Expensive
• Fast	• Slow
• Better for rare diseases	• Better for rare exposures
• Subject to more bias in exposure information	• Subject to more bias in disease diagnosis
• Subject to incomplete data as a result of lack of recall or record	• Subject to incomplete data as a result of loss to follow-up
• Able to provide data on the odds ratio as an estimate of relative risk, but no incidence rates	• Able to provide data on the relative risk, as well as the incidence rates of disease outcome

sifying them by their varying distances from ground zero at the moment of the blast. Occupational cohorts are also very important. For example, all the workers in a pesticide manufacturing plant who were employed there in the same time period might be subdivided into the specific kind of work done and then followed up over time. One famous occupational cohort study examined bus workers to assess the effects of physical work on heart disease rates. On double-decker buses in London, there are two kinds of workers: the drivers, who are sedentary, and the ticket collectors, who are walking up and down the stairs and along the aisles. These workers were presumed to have roughly the same environmental exposures and socioeconomic status and to differ markedly only in whether their job was sedentary.

Another famous cohort study is the Framingham study. In the late

1940s the U.S. Public Health Service decided to follow a large cohort to study the occurrence of cardiovascular disease. A cross-section of socioeconomic, ethnic, occupational, and other demographic groups was desired, so the differences in heart disease rates owing to many factors could be examined. A random sample was selected from Framingham, Massachusetts, a town of about 28,000 people. The original sample was 6,507 people ages 30 to 59, and this was later expanded. Population lists were prepared annually to facilitate sampling and follow-up, and the town's government, hospital, and doctors agreed to participate. To this day, data concerning physical as well as social variables are collected from each participant on an ongoing basis. This huge study requires a large permanent staff.

It's important to keep in mind that a cohort is a clearly defined group. It is often chosen because an organization grants access to data and makes us feel confident of obtaining good follow-up. Therefore, the motivation of volunteer participants and their membership in groups with administrative structures already in place are highly advantageous. Members of the armed forces, medical school alumni associations, and insurance plans are much sought after as participants in cohort studies. Workers at a particular place of employment and labor union members are also much used for this purpose.

INCOMPLETE DATA, LOSS TO FOLLOW-UP, AND OTHER POTENTIAL SOURCES OF BIAS

An important assumption about the cohort is that the individuals who are exposed and are in the study are representative of all those who are exposed in the population in terms of their risk of disease. Likewise, those who are unexposed to the risk factor and are in the study must be representative of the general population who are unexposed in terms of their risk of disease. These assumptions may not always hold in the real world: for example, suppose that some people who work for a company that operates nuclear power plants handle hazardous substances and are considered exposed. Others who work for the same company do administrative or executive work and are considered unexposed. If a minority of the exposed workers volunteer for the study, and they are all the exposed workers with health problems, the rate of illness among the exposed will be overestimated. On the other hand, if the unexposed workers are also differentially likely to volunteer for the study if they have illnesses, not only will their prevailing rate of illness be overestimated, but any real difference between disease rates among the exposed and unexposed might be minimized or undetectable.

The cohort must be determined to be free of the disease under study at the beginning of the study. Then information must be obtained on exposure or other variables affecting disease frequency. This information may be obtained from records or by interview. It may be necessary to have a study staff to conduct medical or other tests on participants or to monitor, say, the environmental conditions prevalent where cohort members live or work. Exposure information that has been recorded by outside parties is particularly desirable, especially if it was recorded before there was knowledge of the disease of interest, helping to exclude the possibility of bias.

Information provided by cohort members concerning exposure may be biased. Individuals may not accurately report their smoking or dietary histories or may be unaware of environmental exposures. They may be motivated by denial to minimize exposure risk, or they may be motivated by anxiety to exaggerate exposure. Still, data on exposure tend to be better in cohort studies than in case-control studies, since the problem of data accuracy is not generally compounded by the problem of data loss over time through failure of memory or loss of records.

Another methodological problem with data from individuals in a cohort is the effect of nonresponse. Nonresponse here refers to nonresponse to inquiries made to obtain information on risks. Over time, cohort members may be sent questionnaires or be asked to undergo a physical examination. A certain proportion may not respond or will fail to provide the desired information and cannot be included in the analysis of study outcomes. Nonresponse has costs in terms of the statistical power of the study, but, more important, it may be differentially biased.

Suppose nonresponse is biased with respect to exposure but not with respect to outcome. Say persons with high levels of radiation exposure refuse to participate in a study of a certain cancer. Our estimated distribution of the group's overall radiation exposure will be biased downward, but ordinarily any association between radiation and the cancer will still be there. Now let's change the scenario. Suppose nonresponse is biased with respect to outcome but not with respect to exposure. Perhaps people with the most advanced cancer can't participate. Assume that nonresponse has no association with radiation exposure level. Then we would underestimate the rates of illness in our sample. The big problem arises if we assume nonresponse to be biased with respect to both illness and exposure. In this scenario, individuals who have both high levels of radiation exposure *and* advanced cancer tend to be nonresponders. Those with high levels of exposure who are left in our sample might tend to be those in whom cancer didn't occur, and our estimate of the association would be affected.

Often, if the nonresponse rate is high, a follow-up effort may be launched involving a resurvey of the nonresponders or even visiting homes or medical institutions to obtain the missing data. This could get expensive. Another way to deal with the problem of nonresponders is to see whether they differ from the original cohort distribution on variables originally recorded that have a bearing on the likelihood of being exposed to the risk factor or having the disease. Age, sex, race, occupation, and exposure levels at the start of the study are often used this way. Distributions of variables in the responding and nonresponding groups are often compared by statistical methods such as chi-square analysis, if the variables are categorical, and *t* tests, if the variables are continuous.

Once the follow-up period of a cohort study has been completed, the determination of outcome must be made for each patient, and the rates of disease in the exposure groups or categories must be compared. Since the usual outcome of interest is morbidity or mortality from a carefully defined disease or group of diseases, the determination of outcome typically depends on such data sources as computerized surveillance of death certificates or hospital admissions or periodic medical examination of each cohort member by a clinical member of the study team. It's important to avoid bias in the ascertainment of disease state, which might occur if the clinician making the assessment knows whether the patient was exposed or not. "Blind" assessment, in which the judge of outcome is unaware of exposure status, is usually best. It's also best to rely on a routinized procedure in which a common protocol for determining disease status is applied equally to all persons in the cohort; this may often be accomplished by searching routine records already kept by an outside party. Typical sources of such records include pension funds, treatment centers, disease registries, insurance plans, and the state. It can happen that some members of the cohort are no longer under the surveillance of the record-keeping agency, because they've emigrated or changed names or occupations, they're no longer covered by the insurance plan, or other similar administrative reasons. Complete and unbiased ascertainment of outcome is an ideal, of course, and one that requires much effort to approach or achieve.

HISTORICAL COHORT STUDIES

In a variant of the cohort study called the *historical cohort study*, researchers use existing records to classify cohorts that started out in the past in terms of their exposure status as of some date or cohort-defining event. The information on the occurrence of disease, which is already present, is traced for these individuals from the time of exposure to the present time. Sometimes follow-up on further occurrence of disease is also conducted. The historical cohort study is conceptually like the cohort studies using concurrent, ongoing data collection, because the study begins with information on a cohort's exposure and examines subsequent disease occurrence. The difference is that the data on exposure classification are from existing records, as are some or all of the data on disease outcome. A number of historical cohort studies are underway and use records from Blue Cross/Blue Shield, Kaiser-Permanente, and other organizations in the health care field. These data sources have the advantage of large sample sizes and long-term collection of data, so that as hypotheses are developed, exposure cohorts can be constructed and subsequent disease rates in the groups can be assessed. However, it is possible that not all diagnoses are equally likely to be accurately reported in these databases.

Disease Rates, Measures of Risk, and Attributable Risk

Some measures of outcome can be calculated from a cohort study that cannot be calculated from a case-control study. The actual *disease rates* in the exposed and unexposed groups (per year or other unit of time) can be obtained for the cohort, because denominators are available representing the persons at risk, among whom the reported cases of disease occurred. Since actual disease rates can be obtained, the relative risk, which is the ratio of the rate among the exposed to the rate among the unexposed, can also be obtained. Recall our earlier discussion of the odds ratio, which is used to estimate relative risk in case-control studies. The relative risk itself is unavailable in such studies, because the rates of disease in the groups are unavailable. When a case-control study is performed, the cases are gathered and compared with controls, but there is no clear denominator from whom these cases are drawn, and it's not known over what period of time disease occurred in them. Cohort studies can tell us rates of disease, and we can see from the rates, using relative risk, that an exposed person is three times more likely than an unexposed person to get a disease. Case-control studies can also tell us, through the odds ratio, that the rate is three times as high among the exposed than among the unexposed, but they can't tell us the actual rate of disease. Just as the null hypothesis for the odds ratio in a case-control study is that the ratio is 1.0, the null hypothesis for the relative risk in a cohort study is that the risk is 1.0. A high level of relative risk indicates that the exposure under study is a powerful etiological agent. In estimating relative risk, we need to guard against the effects of confounding variables. They may be avoided in cohort studies in the same ways they may be avoided in case-control studies; these methods were discussed earlier.

The importance of risk factors for disease outcomes in cohort studies can also be examined by measures of attributable risk. These measures are interpreted in cohort studies in the same way they're interpreted in case-control studies. They are a composite of the risk conferred by an exposure and the prevalence of that exposure in the population and indicate the effect that eliminating a risk factor would have on the overall rate of a disease. A highly risky exposure that affects very few workers may have little impact from a public health point of view, if there are other substantial causes of this illness in the population.

Two of the attributable risk measures that may be obtained from cohort studies are attributable risk in the study population and population attributable risk proportion. *Attributable risk in the study population* is simply the incidence rate in the exposed group minus the incidence rate in the unexposed group. We attribute the difference in rates to the exposure factor under study, on the assumption that other factors responsible for disease or mortality affect our groups equally.

The *population attributable risk proportion* tells you what proportion of disease occurring in the population at large (not the study population) is attributed to exposure, again on the assumption that other factors responsible for disease affect the exposed and unexposed segments of the general population equally. This measure is calculated by (1) obtaining the rates of disease in the exposed and the unexposed groups in the study population, (2) dividing the general population into exposed and unexposed groups, (3) applying the corresponding groups' disease rates from the study population to the numbers of persons in these groups in the general population, and (4) determining how many cases (per thousand or other round number) would be eliminated if all of the general population were in the unexposed group.

A Word about Terminology

I've consistently used the unambiguous terms *case-control studies* and *cohort studies* in the above discussion, but you should be aware that the terminology used in the medical literature to refer to these types of studies is sometimes confusing. Case-control studies are also sometimes called *retrospective studies*, because they're retrospective in the logical sense that they start with information on the outcome and look backward to ascertain exposure histories among cases and controls. Cohort studies are sometimes called *prospective studies*, because they start with groups sorted according to the presence or absence of a supposed risk factor and examine what happens later in a logical sequence over time: does disease develop or not? There is the potential for confusion, because sometimes historical cohort studies are called *retrospective cohort studies* or even occasionally just *retrospective studies*, a term other authors use to refer exclusively to case-control studies. When you read a medical journal article, however, you should be able to tell what has been done in terms of follow-up or the examination of records of exposure and disease.

Comparison of the Different Epidemiological Study Designs

The different epidemiological study designs have different advantages and disadvantages. Sometimes a case-control study design may be used because it is generally less expensive and faster than a cohort study. Sometimes a cohort study is performed because rates of illness are desired. Note that when a disease is rare, it may be best to use a case-control study. If a disease occurs in 1 in 10,000 persons in the general population, it may not be practical to accumulate and follow a cohort of the size needed to detect a doubling of risk due to a certain exposure. Investigators may be better off going to a registry of cases of that disease or to a referral hospital that handles many cases. On the other hand, when an exposure is rare, it may be a practical necessity to conduct a cohort study. If exposure to a certain chemical occurs only in the course of a particular industrial process, which few people are involved with, it makes little sense to accumulate cases and controls in the hope that you'll be lucky enough to get some cases with that occupational exposure. Differences in exposure rates between cases and controls may not be detectable. In such a circumstance, a study involving an occupational cohort is more suitable.

Five

Clinical Trials

A clinical trial may be understood as a particular type of cohort study. The exposure of interest is the treatment group, and the outcome is the therapeutic effect, which we usually hope is significantly superior in a certain group or groups. At the start of the clinical trial, everyone is comparable in terms of illness. Medical follow-up, concurrent with treatment (and even afterwards), is used to determine the effects of the treatment.

For the clinician, a clinical trial is an experiment on a sample of patients. It's conducted to permit inference concerning the most suitable treatment of the population of similar patients. For millennia, people have understood that the judgment of whether a therapeutic regimen is safe and effective must be made on the basis of comparative empirical evidence concerning the results of different treatments (or no treatment at all). In ancient Greece, Herodotus reported that people of an even earlier culture, the Babylonians, had the practice of exhibiting sick persons in public squares. People who had had the disease and recovered, or those who had treated it in others, offered their advice to the afflicted. The earliest recorded comparative clinical trial is said to be an account of a clinical trial in two groups that appears in the Book of Daniel in the Hebrew bible. However, early clinical trials such as that one were fraught with problems such as inadequate statistical power and biased assessment of outcome. It has been only in the second half of the twentieth century, with the rise of the theory of hypothesis testing and other principles derived from probability mathematics, that well-designed

Phases of Clinical Trials of New Drugs

An investigational new drug (IND) application gets FDA approval.

Phase I Clinical Trial

- Participants are normal healthy human volunteers.
- All participants receive the new prospective medication.
- The trial produces data on the drug's safety, tolerance, and disposition.
- The trial is often retricted to male subjects.
- Subjects usually number 75 to 150.

Phase II Clinical Trial

- Participants are patients with the target disease.
- Some patients receive a control (a placebo or an existing drug).
- The trial produces data on the drug's safety, tolerance, and efficacy.
- The trial may include studies to find dosage ranges.
- Usually, 500 to 1,000 patients are involved.

Phase III Clinical Trial

- Participants are patients with the target disease.
- Some patients receive a control (a placebo or an existing drug).
- The trial produces the best premarketing data on the drug's safety and efficacy.
- Usually, 1,500 to 5,000 patients are involved.

A new drug application (NDA) gets FDA approval.

Ongoing postmarketing surveillance is conducted
for rare adverse reactions.

clinical trials have become common. Despite the early embrace of the importance of experiment in general by medical scientists, clinical trials in the past that could meet today's standards of rigor were the exception rather than the rule. Pasteur's test of an anthrax vaccine for sheep in the late 1800s was one such exception.

Controls and Placebos

A key element in a good clinical trial is the presence of one or more control groups. Controls enable us to make comparisons between treatments. Sometimes an old treatment is the control: in this case, the existing standard treatment is used to determine whether a novel therapy is more or less advantageous. Sometimes the control is a *placebo*, a pharmacologically inert substance that is substituted for the active treatment. A placebo may be a pill made to look like the active treatment, or it may be an injection of normal saline instead of a solution containing the active ingredient under study.

Placebo is Latin for "I will please," and indeed many placebos are pleasing: administration of a placebo may result in the *placebo effect*, whereby the pharmacologically inactive substance has a real, measurable, objective physiological effect. The magnitude and exact mechanism of placebo effects vary from study to study, but the effects are quite real and may be marked. For example, in a 6-week clinical trial of a diuretic antihypertensive agent, one group received the new agent and another group received a placebo. Patients did not know which group they were in, but they knew they would be receiving either the drug or the placebo. The placebo control group enjoyed a decrease in systolic blood pressure of 5 mmHg, just because they believed they might be receiving an active treatment.

Naturally, the more subjective measures are the most susceptible to the placebo effect. For example, it is not surprising that minor dermatitis responds to placebo to a degree we would not expect in retinoblastoma. After all, perhaps the former condition has a substantial emotional component and is exacerbated by stress, and receiving even a placebo is naturally soothing to the mind. Also, knowing they're under treatment, patients may scratch less and avoid worsening their condition. But even less subjective measures, such as the time to the complete healing of a fracture, as seen on radiography, or the resolution of an infection, have been shown to be beneficially affected by adjunct therapy with placebos. Since the placebo effect is real, when a claim is being made for the effects of a new drug, it is important that those effects exceed the effects induced by the administration of a placebo. Also, undesirable medical events may happen to some patients as the trial proceeds, and some of these events occur at random and not because of the treatment. Use of a placebo group provides a baseline for rates of adverse events that would be expected even in the absence of pharmacological activity.

In some circumstances the administration of a placebo is clearly unethical. For example, if it is well known that an existing standard treatment is vastly more effective than a placebo, it's unethical to withhold the standard treatment and administer a placebo as a control when testing new treatments. When such ethical issues arise, the regulatory agencies that require clinical trials data before they will license a new medicine generally allow (or require) experimenters to forgo placebo controls and use active controls.

Randomization and Assignment to Treatment Groups

Assignment to treatment groups must be random in order for the results of statistical comparisons between groups to be valid. Remember that the statistical tests described in Chapter 2 all produce P values as the result of certain calculations. These calculations all involve random samples. Thanks to statistical tests, we can determine the probability that we would see a sample as odd as ours in terms of its proportions, or its mean value, or the presence of a linear trend, or some other aspect of interest. But when we do the calculations we're always assuming that we're sampling from a distribution consistent with the null hypothesis and that we're examining a random sample from that distribution. The calculations tell us the probability that our observations occurred by chance alone, in the absence of a treatment effect, and this probability will not be correct if the samples are not random.

Randomization helps to ensure that high- and low-risk patients end up equally in the treatment group(s). This means that statistical tests comparing the results of treatments are comparisons between samples of patients who are quite comparable and differ only because of chance fluctuation and possibly the effects of the drug treatment group. They are random samples drawn from the world of possible patients who might get assigned drug A and drug B, and so statistical tests are valid.

This should make intuitive sense to the experimenter who is not a statistician. If assignment to two treatment groups is random, then on average both patients who are extremely sick and would die anyway and patients whose conditions, unbeknownst to the physician, are benign and about to resolve end up equally in the two groups. Nonresponders to drug A end up equally in the two groups, and so do nonresponders to drug B. This makes comparison more purely a comparison between the effects of A and B, with all else equal.

The failure of the Lanarkshire milk experiment in Great Britain in the 1930s demonstrates what can happen if randomization is not followed. The effects of the provision of milk to schoolchildren were the subject of the experiment: would the milk result in any improvement in growth compared to children who did not receive the benefit of this government intervention? Children in various schools were randomized to receive or not receive the supplementary milk. However, some teachers felt sorry for the smaller, slower growing children and ignored the randomization, making their own selection of who ought to receive it. They differentially selected the smaller children, singling them out to receive the milk. Those receiving the milk were disproportionately the children who grew slowly, and they grew slowly for a whole variety of reasons, of course, not just because of dietary insufficiency of a sort that could be corrected by the added milk. Since the slowest growing children ended up in the milk supplementation group, they depressed the measures of growth in that group, and the comparison showed little difference between those who received milk and those who did not. Since the milk supplementation program would have been applied to the general population of children, a better comparison would have been obtained if two random samples from the general population of schoolchildren had been compared, one receiving the milk and one not. Those who wouldn't have benefited in any case from the supplementation ended up disproportionately taking it, obscuring the supplementation's effect.

Sometimes randomization to inactive or even to standard treatments is not acceptable to patients, who insist on trying an experimental therapy. Patients always have the right to be thoroughly informed about experimentation and to refuse to take part in it. Not surprisingly, patients in end-stage disease, for example those with certain cancers, who have no really useful therapeutic options and are desperate to try anything, are especially unwilling to accept placebo. Some limited descriptive knowledge can be gained about the effects of a new treatment under such circumstances, particularly about toxic effects that may be quite expected and that would pose unacceptable risks in other circumstances. Also, it is possible to examine patient progress and compare it with historical controls, that is, with what has generally been seen in untreated patients under the same circumstances. Occasionally, truly remarkable and unexpected clinical efficacy is observed with novel treatments in such patients, although the finding is often anecdotal and not statistically valid evidence. More often, it is unclear what effects the treatment has, perhaps because the acceptance of very risky new treatments without a controlled experiment is generally limited to patients with advanced disease, in whom no treatment might reasonably be expected to have an effect. In consequence, perhaps some treatments that would be of therapeutic value in patients with less advanced disease go unremarked because they're tested only in patients for whom death is imminent.

Adaptive Allocation and Stopping Rules

The clinician should be aware of several variant procedures that pertain to treatment assignment. One is adaptive allocation. *Adaptive allocation* means that a patient coming in is assigned to a treatment group based in part on how the therapeutic effects of the treatments compare thus far in the trial. The allocation is decided according to complex rules of probability in order to maximize the chance that a significant difference will be found. This provides the ethical advantage that each patient is subjected to the minimum risk of taking an ineffective substance, as judged by the current state of knowledge at the time of his or her entry to the trial.

A variety of *stopping rules* have also been devised to permit ending a clinical trial as soon as possible to allow patients on the less effective therapy to be transferred to the more effective one as soon as possible. Like adaptive allocation, this has ethical advantages and may also incorporate the ongoing acquisition of knowledge about the therapy as the trial proceeds, so that the trial may be stopped as soon as adequate evidence in support of the null hypothesis or its alternative is shown.

Cross-over Designs

Finally, in *cross-over designs* each patient takes each of the (usually two) treatments. The treatment groups differ with respect to the order of the treatments. For example, if we're testing drugs A and B, one group receives drug A first and then drug B. For the other group the order is reversed. Sometimes there is a *washout period* between the administrations of the two treatments. The advantage to this method is that each patient serves as his or her own control, and the effect of interindividual variability is minimized. However, this method can't always be used, because it rests on the assumption that there is no carryover effect of the first treatment during the second treatment period.

Other Types of Randomized Trials

Randomization is not limited to pharmaceutical trials, of course. As an example, I participated in the evaluation of a clinical trial of orthopedic procedures for fixing ankle fractures. The orthopedist believed that his new method shortened the time the patient spent on the operating table and subjected the patient to less insult, since fewer fixators were used; he also believed that healing time would improve compared to the standard method and that joint stability would be the same. A comparison was called for. Patients were randomized as they came in with the clinical problem, receiving, with equal probability, either one treatment or the other. Randomization in surgery clinical trials is not uncommon.

In practice, randomization is usually accomplished by computer programs. Some randomization schemes are quite complex. For example, patients are randomized within blocks, first to one treatment and then another, to ensure representation of patients within treatment groups. The calculation methods for P values must take into account the randomization method used.

"Blind" Assessment of Trial Outcomes

Clinical trials are often conducted in what is termed a *blind* (or, to use a more genteel term, *masked*) fashion. *Double-blind* trials are common. In a double-blind trial, neither the patient nor those responsible for the patient's clinical evaluation know which treatment he or she is receiving. This way, bias is avoided: the patient's response cannot be influenced by his or her faith or lack of faith in the assigned treatment. Similarly, the health care worker assessing the patient will make observations and recommendations and evaluate therapeutic effects objectively, since there cannot be any prior expectation as to the effects of a treatment that may be novel, standard, or inert.

Efforts to avoid bias in clinical trials are important, because it is known that patients may report faster progress if they believe they've been selected to receive a new treatment, even one that later turns out to have no therapeutic value and is toxic. Similarly, it has been documented that physicians, on average, report faster resolution of medical problems when the patient is on a therapy they believe in. These biases are more pronounced when there is a greater subjectivity in the assessment of outcome. Self-reported severity of headache may be more biased than a measure such as wheal size in the patient population. A physician may be more prone to bias when assessing a rash than when assessing forced expiratory volume. But biases may exist in almost any measurement, and it's better to guard against them than to find out later that there has been a major expenditure for a flawed clinical trial. Of course, blinding is not always a practical possibility. For example, it may be evident to both the patient and the physician which external fixator was used to correct an orthopedic problem.

Consent and the Ethics of Human Experimentation

Some people believe that clinical trials are unethical and ask, "How can you deny patients the latest in medical treatment?" The person asking such a question makes the implicit assumption that a new treatment is better than an old treatment, in terms of improved therapeutic efficacy and fewer side effects. This is not always the case, however. The reasonable expectation from lab evidence that a compound will be useful in treating people isn't proof; it's just a hypothesis. Sometimes the hypothesis is correct, and sometimes it's grossly incorrect. It's the job of the clinical trialist to test the hypothesis by experiment. In the late 1940s and early 1950s, it was considered obvious that premature infants with poorly developed lungs would benefit from being placed in an atmosphere of pure oxygen. An experiment, it was thought, would delay implementation of this useful therapeutic regimen and was totally unnecessary. A totally unforeseen result of this treatment, however, was a condition called retrolental fibroplasia, which caused blindness in thousands of newborns subjected to the oxygen atmosphere.

In fact, an experiment is performed every time a new treatment is put into use, even when the use of the treatment is not sanctioned by the scientific establishment but occurs "underground," that is, in times and places where medicines are not examined by the government for proof of safety and efficacy. The question is, How is knowledge going to be gathered, analyzed, and disseminated from the inevitable experiment? Perhaps knowledge is going to be gained in a systematic way that excludes the problems described above, which, if left unchecked, would wreak havoc on the comparability of treatment groups. This is the way of the clinical trial. Alternatively, perhaps data will be made available in a haphazard and largely unrecorded fashion from an experiment that had poor controls, was fraught with biases, and doesn't permit useful comparisons with other treatments.

The perpetual pressure to bring drugs through clinical trials more quickly is warranted, because people are suffering during the time it takes to perform a controlled experiment. If a drug works, the time needed to demonstrate that fact experimentally may delay the availability of the drug to people who need it, with real adverse consequences. But if a drug doesn't work, and has side effects, regulatory agencies are not doing patients any favor by letting it be marketed at all, and are causing even more harm by accelerating its availability. Unfortunately, the clinical trial is the most scientifically valid way to assess whether a drug works or not, for all the reasons given above, and one of the tragedies of life is that while the information is slowly being gathered, people are suffering. Yet researchers must gather that information carefully and systematically, for if they are not required to do so, harmful drugs may be put on the market. Political, social, and economic means must be found to accelerate the discovery and validation of new therapies to minimize the human cost of this dilemma.

Nevertheless, some people still continue to feel appalled at the idea of patients' being randomized to treatments in an experiment, or think that a double-blind experiment is a ghastly idea. By law, no person can compel another to submit to a medical experiment, no matter what importance the medical community attaches to the study and no matter what the biostatistical community says about the perfection of the study design. All clinical trials in the United States must be approved by an institutional review board, whose composition ordinarily includes scientists and clinical personnel, members of the clergy, and members of the public. Other countries require the approval of similar panels. For pharmaceutical trials, most countries also require approval by government regulatory agencies before a clinical trial can begin. This approval is generally based on scientific and ethical criteria. Clinical trials of surgical or radiological treatments do not require regulatory approval in all countries, but they do require approval of a body akin to the institutional review board in most countries, including the United States. These boards require that informed consent be signed by the patient indicating that various aspects of the study, including, where relevant, randomization to treatments and the use of a single- or double-blind procedure, have been explained.

A controversial change has recently been made in the United States: in some circumstances where the patient is typically unconscious and next of kin are typically unavailable to give permission, informed consent may not be required. An example of such circumstances is severe traumatic injury, where the treatment under study must be applied during the first few hours of care in an emergency room in hopes of preventing brain injury. Such protocols would still require board approval before an experiment could be undertaken.

The inherently uncertain nature of medical knowledge has caused many false starts and mistaken approaches to therapy over the centuries. In recent times, it has become possible to quantify the reliability of inferences from experimental observations. This quantification has been made possible by the recognition of certain assumptions and the concomitant application of laws of probability, which have a bearing on random error. Clinicians have not only come to understand the necessity of reasoning probabilistically, but have begun to accumulate the tools to do so. These tools include a wide variety of statistical tests, as well as statistically valid techniques for designing epidemiological studies and clinical trials. In the final analysis, the world of medical science in general will gain much from statistically valid study design. Perhaps the late Lewis Thomas, a distinguished scientist and writer and the physician-in-chief at Memorial Sloan-Kettering Cancer Center, said it best. As he put it, "Hunches and intuitive impressions are essential for getting the work started, but it is only through the quality of the numbers at the end that the truth can be told."

Additional Reading

Bailar, J. C., and Mosteller, F. *Medical Uses of Statistics*. Boston: New England Journal of Medicine Books, 1992. A wide variety of issues concerning the appropriate collection and interpretation of medical statistics is discussed thoroughly. The topics and mathematical level are well suited to a medical audience. Subjects I haven't covered in the present book are treated, such as meta-analysis, how to use a statistical consultant, and further topics in survival analysis. This book is a good resource for the clinician who needs to interpret published medical literature.

Campbell, M. J., and Machin, D. *Medical Statistics: A Commonsense Approach*. 2d ed. New York: John Wiley & Sons, 1993. This clearly written book presents numerous common statistical methods and includes appendices showing calculation procedures. Tables of statistical values needed for the interpretation of results are also provided for a few of the more commonly used distributions. This book is very useful to the clinician who is starting in research.

Hamming, R. W. *The Art of Probability for Scientists and Engineers*. New York: Addison-Wesley, 1991. In this beautifully written book, Hamming explains the laws of probability and how they can be used to model empirical scientific realities. He draws heavily on common experiences and the reader's quantitative intuition; the mathematical level is limited essentially to tools of elementary algebra and scant calculus. Although this book isn't a statistics book, it elegantly systematizes and quantifies the scientific reader's approach to probability.

Hennekens, C. H., and Buring, J. E. *Epidemiology in Medicine.* Boston: Little, Brown, 1987. Aimed at a wide physician audience, this book is a good, in-depth treatment of study design issues in epidemiology.

Kendall, M. G., and Stuart, A. *The Advanced Theory of Statistics.* New York: Hafner, 1966. This book requires a thorough grounding in mathematics; it provides rigorous demonstrations of the validity of statistical tests and provides the mathematically sophisticated reader with a framework permitting the development of new statistical tools.

Kraemer, H. C., and Thiemann, S. *How Many Subjects? Statistical Power Analysis in Research.* Newbury Park, Calif.: Sage, 1987. Instructions on calculating power for a variety of statistical methods, such as chi-square, correlation, and regression, are given. These calculations cannot be accomplished without mathematical treatment, but this introduction is the simplest I know of. Because the book is written for a social science audience, some of the examples may not seem relevant, but the medical person who wants a book on how to do power calculations would do well to start with this one.

Le, C. T., and Boen, J. R. *Health and Numbers: Basic Biostatistical Methods.* New York: Wiley-Liss, 1995. Like Campbell and Machin's book, this is a clearly written presentation of a number of the more common statistical tests and how to perform them, though perhaps the mathematical level of this one is a bit lower and fewer methods are presented. Tables of statistical values needed for the interpretation of results are provided for a few commonly used distributions. This is a good first book with equations for a medical student or the novice physician-researcher.

Lilienfeld, D. E., and Stolley, P. D. *Foundations of Epidemiology.* 3d ed. New York: Oxford University Press, 1994. This is a revision of a classic and thorough introduction to epidemiological and clinical trials study designs.

Murphy, E. A. *Probability in Medicine.* Baltimore: Johns Hopkins University Press, 1979. For the most part, only high school algebra is needed to read and understand this book, but it's still not a book for the math phobic: equations abound, and the orientation is toward the development of mathematical models of such clinically relevant matters as the life spans of blood platelets. To gain insight from this book, the reader must attentively work through the examples and the problems. However, the effort is richly repaid. This volume is a superb introduction for the clinical researcher working in such fields as physiology and genetics.

Smith, C. G. *The Process of New Drug Discovery and Development.* Boca Raton, Fla.: CRC Press, 1992. This is a nontechnical book by someone who worked both as a scientist and as a senior executive in several corporations in the pharmaceutical industry. Smith offers a succinct treatment of the entire process of drug discovery and development, including screening of new compounds; studies of toxicology, metabolism, and drug disposition; initial experiments on people; and the roles of biometrics and computerization in drug studies. The book is an excellent overview for someone working for the first time on the development of new drugs.

Weaver, W. *Lady Luck: The Theory of Probability.* New York: Dover, 1982. Using only prose, just a bit of arithmetic, and no higher mathematics, Weaver treats a variety of topics in probability theory in a useful and understandable way. The binomial theorem, the law of large numbers, Chebychev's theorem, and the concept of a distribution function are all clearly and accurately explained. This book is accessible for anyone in science or medicine, although the examples are from all fields and from everyday life.

Index